I0091271

HEALING WITH
FLOWER ESSENCES

*How to Use Natural Botanicals
for Spiritual and Emotional Well-Being*

HEALING WITH FLOWER ESSENCES

*How to Use Natural Botanicals
for Spiritual and Emotional Well-Being*

Joan Greenblatt

■■ Aperion Books
www.AperionBooks.com

APERION BOOKS™
1611A S. Melrose Dr. #173
Vista, California 92081
www.AperionBooks.com

Copyright © 2011 by Joan Greenblatt
www.EssentialFlowerRemedies.com

All rights reserved. No part of this book may be reproduced or transmitted in any form or by any means, electronic or mechanical, including photocopying, recordings, or by any information storage and retrieval system, without written permission from the author, except for the inclusion of a brief quotation in a review.

First Edition 2011
Printed in the United States of America

ISBN-10: 0-0829678-0-2
ISBN-13: 978-0-9829678-0-5

Library of Congress Catalog Card Number: 2010912742

Cover & book design by CenterPointe Media
www.CenterPointeMedia.com

Always consult your doctor for any and all medical conditions. This book is not intended to diagnose, treat, cure, or prevent any disease. Flower Essences are never meant as a replacement or substitute for any type of medical treatment.

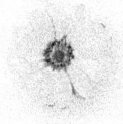

DEDICATION

This book is dedicated to Lucy, my first flower
essence teacher, who showed me how to live in the
world while catching the spirit within. She will
always be a source of inspiration.

To my husband and daughter, who never
cease to amaze me with their unbounded
encouragement and love. They both endured years
of probing and experimentation.

To my dear parents, who have always been
a steady and loving support.

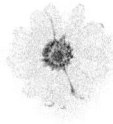

ACKNOWLEDGEMENTS

First and foremost, I must acknowledge the flower essences themselves: they speak to me everyday—and when I am receptive, I am able to hear their profound messages.

I greatly honor my second flower essence mentor, Jan Kalmbach, who led me through the meadow of flowers with grace and insight.

I offer grateful thanks to those who have been on this journey with me throughout the years of compiling this book, and whose encouragement and love are always with me: Chetna Bhatt, Nancy Copen, and Phyllis Kahaney. Special thanks to Terrin Irwin, my proofreader, who offered many helpful organizational tips.

I couldn't have accomplished this without my husband's editing. Matthew went through the manuscript's many incarnations, always bringing great depth, while prodding me to self-edit and enhance the chapters by adding practical tools.

And also much gratitude goes to my clients and friends, who I continue to work with over the years. They teach me that although our challenges appear differently, we are all the same essence.

May we walk toward happiness—our innate nature—
in all that we do.

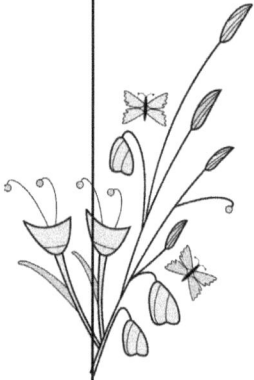

"If you know you are alive,

find the essence of life.

Life is the sort of guest

you don't meet twice.

A drop melting into the sea

Everyone can see.

But the sea absorbed in a drop

only a rare one can follow!

To see a world in a grain of sand,

And a heaven in a wild flower,

Hold infinity in the palm of your hand,

And eternity in an hour."

—WILLIAM BLAKE

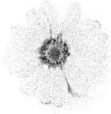

CONTENTS

INTRODUCTION

Chapter One
THE ESSENCE OF FLOWERS

Chapter Eight
FLOWER ESSENCE STUDIES

Chapter Nine
THE FLOWER ESSENCE KITCHEN

Chapter Ten
CONCLUSION

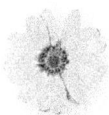

INTRODUCTION

"Where flowers bloom so does hope."
LADY BIRD JOHNSON

THE HEALING POWER OF FLOWER ESSENCES

An interesting subtitle for this book could have been "Sunshine Wattle and the Power of Flowers." When I first caught a glimpse of the "Dr. Seuss-looking" Sunshine Wattle, it was love at first sight. You could call this flower a "Zen essence," since it nudges us toward unconditional acceptance of the beauty and joy in the present moment. It is these very qualities that flower essences help to restore in us that inspired me to write this book. Flower essences hold within them the remarkable energetic power of healing at the cellular level and, as a result, can change lives in dramatic ways. As a complementary, energetic healing therapy, flowers and their potent essences hold a vital key for the challenges we face in the world today.

"The voyage of discovery is not in seeking new landscapes, but in having new eyes."
–MARCEL PROUST

"People do not weave the web of life; they are merely a strand in it. Whatever one does to the web, one does to oneself."
—CHIEF SEATTLE

Although this book isn't meant to be an anthology of flower essences, the last chapter does contain valuable reference materials which includes: 84 flower essence descriptions, 13 aromatherapeutic extracts, an alphabetized index, diagnosis form, and a dosage guide.

The spirit of this book is meant to awaken you, the reader, to a sense of wonder at nature's healing gifts that grow wild in far-flung fields and in our own backyards. As a collective village, we may overlook what is most obvious, especially the humble flowers that grow around us. Shining a light on the healing power of flower essences will hopefully give you an opportunity to open to its life-affirming possibilities.

I've changed the names of the people that I've worked with to protect their privacy. However, their stories are accurate and have been documented to inspire and instruct. By including diagnostic tools, exercises, and checklists, my sincere hope is that the healing power of flowers will speak to you and that you will be inspired to try them for yourself. To round out the presentation, I've added a number of inspiring quotes that I collected over many years. This book is dedicated to sharing a sense of wonder and joy through words and the silence that surrounds them.

"In the cherry blossom's shade;
there's no such thing as a stranger."
—KOBAYASHI ISSA

REDISCOVERING AN OLD FRIEND

It was a long, chilly, gray spring day—the kind that we seemed to experience for two months running. A rolling mist from the Bay of Fundy hugged the North Mountain like the frothy foam on top of a latté. So when the clouds finally dissipated a little and the sun broke through the bits of blue sky, I felt as if I were born again. My first few months of living in a meditation center on the peninsula of Nova Scotia, Canada, left me hungering for the brief, but ecstatic summer months that were to come and go in the blink of an eye. I was in my early twenties during that first summer of discovery, and in those warm, bright Acadian days, my fascination with flowers began. It felt as if I was rediscovering a long-lost, treasured friend. I remember the exact moment, too.

"We must never cease from exploration. And the end of all our exploring will be to arrive where we began and to know the place for the first time."
–T. S. ELIOT

"Little things seem nothing, but they give peace, like those meadow flowers which individually seem odorless but all together perfume the air."
—GEORGES BERNANOS

The old farmhouse we lived in sat at the base of a mountain located in the Annapolis Valley, the verdant land sandwiched between the North and South Mountain range

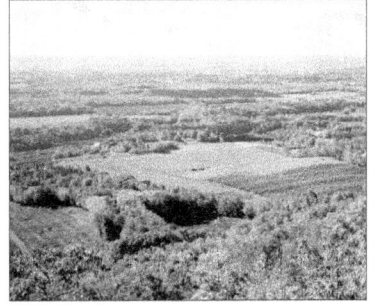

A view of the Annapolis Valley from a lookout on the top of the North Mountain.

(running 93 miles along the Bay of Fundy coast). In fact, the property went right up to the North Mountain's summit. When I ventured out that first time and began to walk up the mountain, a meadow suddenly appeared as if out of nowhere. Why this area of land didn't accommodate the evergreen forest that grew on every other patch of land on the mountain will always puzzle me. When I reached the meadow on that spring morning, the blanket of wildflowers took my breath away. I soon discovered the proud, delicate blossom of a few pink Lady's Slippers. Later I found out how rare they were, and that one should absolutely not pick them, as they need to cycle through the seasons to regenerate themselves. But at the time it was just a pretty pink flower. I also found the curiously named Goatsbeard, which I first thought was a dandelion, but upon further inspection noticed the leaves to be different, and its cousin Devil's Paintbrush, which was a brilliant orange. The green Solomon's Seal, with its arching stems and feathery, creamy-white mass of tiny flowers, were growing in the shaded areas along the edge of the meadow. The list (whose names and properties I discovered later on in my research) goes on. I sat amongst them, felt their healing power, and heard their gentle voices. I wondered about their existence: what birds had dropped the first seeds on this small but fertile meadow, hidden deep within the densely, forested mountain.

"Many eyes go through the meadow, but few see the flowers in it."
–RALPH WALDO EMERSON

"When you are inspired by some great purpose, some extraordinary project, all your thoughts break their bonds; your mind transcends limitations, your consciousness expands in every direction, and you find yourself in a new, great, and wonderful world."
—PATANJALI

It all began that morning—the wonder, delight, and fascination with flowers amidst the silence and harmony of nature. Later, I was to learn that others, especially the pioneers who discovered the healing properties of plants, often experienced it in a similar way. During that brief morning of "flower meditation," I knew that I had touched upon the mystery and majesty of an ancient world, and it opened me up to its limitless possibilities.

"If you want to make your dreams come true,
the first thing you have to do is wake up."
—J. M. POWER

Eight years later, my husband Matthew and I found ourselves in South India working on a special publication, I was the designer and

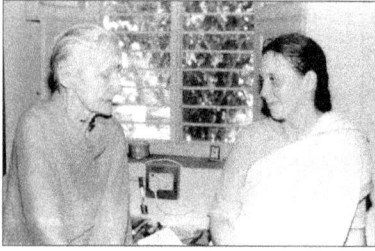

Lucy and Joan

Matthew was editor of the project. It was in this ancient land that I first discovered Bach Flower Essences. A German mystic, Lucy Cornelssen, was a dear friend and teacher, and I visited with her often. Her quiet dignity and peaceful presence drew me to her again and again. One day, I saw her take a vial from an end-table drawer and put two drops from it onto her tongue. She saw my questioning look and instead of telling me what she had just taken, she handed me a well-worn book and told me to read it. It was an Indian edition of a book on Bach Flower Essences. I devoured the book; it was a revelation to me, and a clear understanding of something I intuitively knew to be true.

"Creativity involves breaking out of established patterns
in order to look at things in a different way."
—EDWARD DE BONO

The next time I met Lucy, she greeted me with a wide smile; she knew that I knew. We then began a journey of flower essence discovery. She told me how the remedies had kept her vital even into her nineties. One by one, we went through each remedy. We first visited with the wispy *Clematis*, that helped clear the sleepy-headed, confused, pie-in-the-sky emotional type. Being a visual learner, I formed a picture in my mind of this initial essence and dubbed it, "Lucy in the Sky with Diamonds." Doing this made it easier for me to remember each distinctive character trait. The essence Lucy often used herself was the loopy and hardy *White Chestnut*. This essence calms the flow of thoughts that revolves in endless circles. Lucy described it as the "escalator essence." She said it calmed her mind and soothed her heart!

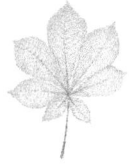

Our publication project took nearly two years to complete, and throughout that time I mentored with Lucy, beginning my lifelong experimentation with flower essences.

Lucy also spoke to me about developing an inner guide in order to use this understanding to help others. She often said that "conscious listening" consists of not only listening to the words of others, but also to the space between the words too. She pointed out that listening nonjudgementally and without interference allows the person to feel safe and open. It is in this openness that feelings and issues can be expressed and the appropriate healing essence revealed.

A few months later, shortly after investing in a set of flower essences, a remarkable incident took place. One morning, I witnessed a little kitten being viciously attacked by a stray dog. The kitten lay lifeless in front of our cottage and was unresponsive to our touch. I was sure it had either not survived or was gravely injured. Not knowing what else to do, I placed a few drops of *Rescue Remedy*® in the kitten's mouth. Within a few moments, I was astounded to see the kitten fully wake, shake its head, and, in a dazed manner, simply bound away.

The incident with the kitten marked the beginning of my journey to help people I would meet along life's path. One of my first cases was a young man, Michael, who had travelled to India to get through the devastating loss of his newly married wife. She had died a short time after they were married. One morning, she simply didn't wake up. In the year that followed her sudden death, Michael tried everything to reconnect with life but the wound was too deep, too raw. So, he thought a change of place may help. Of course, it didn't because he brought his mind and the emotional pain that still

White Chestnut Leaf

"The first step toward change is acceptance. Once you accept yourself, you open the door to change.

Change is not something you do, it's something you allow."

—WILL GARCIA

lived within it with him. Michael spoke about his feelings of guilt and extreme emptiness; he blamed himself for not being able to do anything to help her that morning. The "roar of guilt" was deafening and absorbed any ability he had to move on. So, along with a few other essences, the stately *Pine* (an essence that helps one stop holding onto guilt) was in order. I gave him a bottle of combination drops and waited. I didn't have to wait long. Within days there was a new spring in his step, a noticeable relaxation upon his face, and almost a smile . . . almost. Then, a week later, I passed him on the street and I noticed on his face a full-on grin. At that moment I knew he was starting to accept his new reality and to embrace life again.

> *"We have more possibilities available in*
> *each moment than we realize."*
> —THICH NHAT HANH

Many instances like Michael's have taken place through the decades of working with flower essences. Over time, I learned about other flower essence systems and eventually took advanced courses from accredited organizations that offer flower essence practitioner diploma programs. I soon began to add a variety of essences to my répertoire and found that specific combinations offered profound, subtle, and spiritual results.

As I studied flower essences more deeply, especially their origins and applications in different parts of the world, I became more awe-inspired. It was clear that the emotional challenges that are part of the human experience also hold within them the seeds of their own natural cures. Flowers, with their powerful healing abilities, were simply waiting for us in the exalted Himalayan mountaintops, growing in outcrops upon the rugged Alaskan landscape, lifting their heads amid the arid and dry Australian outback, basking in the pristine English countryside, and covering the sunlit Californian meadows.

> *It never ceases to amaze me that nature has all the answers;*
> *we only have to listen closely to its whisper.*

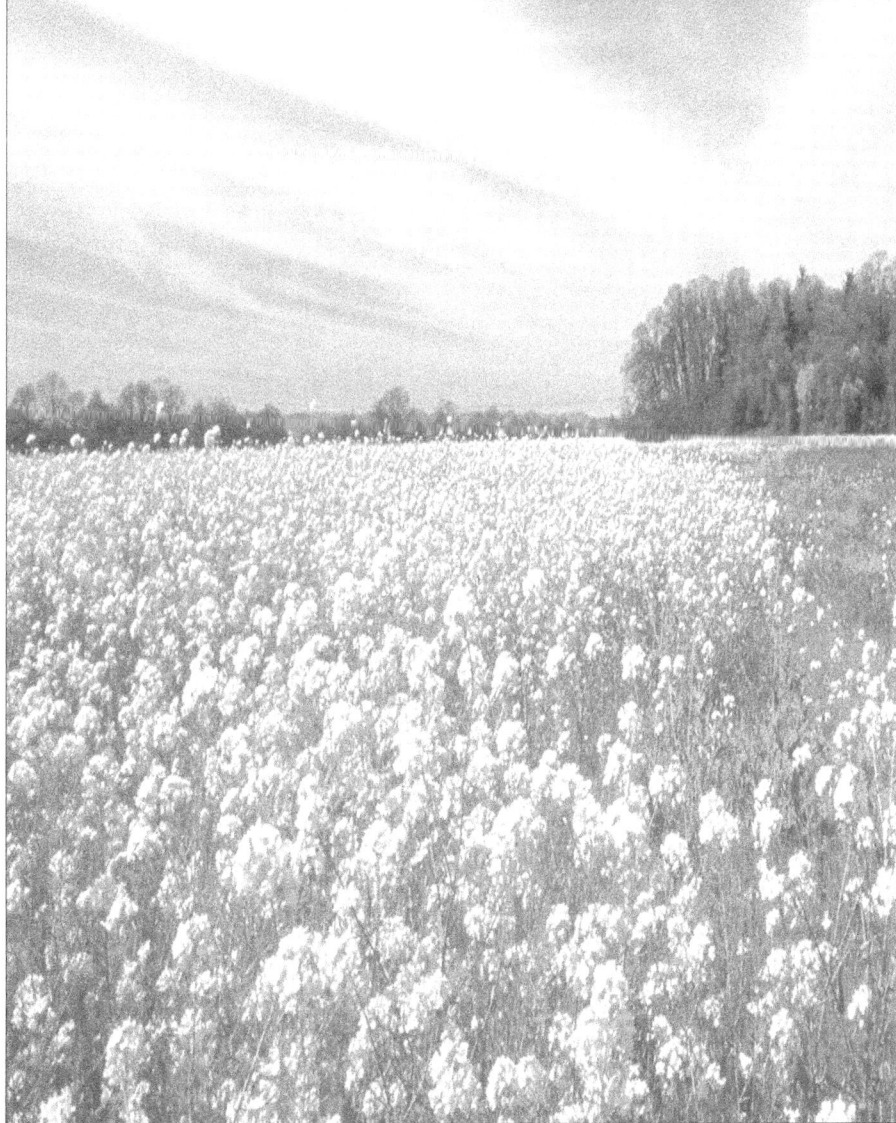

"The temple bell stops but I still hear the sound coming out of the flowers."
—Matsuo Basho

*"Flowers . . . are a proud assertion
that a ray of beauty outvalues
all the utilities of the world."*
—RALPH WALDO EMERSON

*"Just living is not enough . . . one
must have sunshine, freedom,
and a little flower."*
—HANS CHRISTIAN ANDERSON

"Wisdom begins in wonder."
—SOCRATES

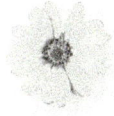

Chapter One

THE ESSENCE OF FLOWERS

*"Flowers always make people better, happier and more helpful;
they are sunshine, food, and medicine to the soul."*
—LUTHER BURBANK

SUBTLE ENERGY

Flower essences contain nature's vibrational energy. They hold within them a healing balm that allows our emotional issues, blocks, and challenges to find a pathway to peace and resolve. Oftentimes, we mask emotional challenges behind physical discomfort. A stomachache may be the result of long-held stress or repression of a true feeling; a blinding headache may mask fear, trauma, or loss. The combinations are as endless as are individuals. Ailments such as backaches, low energy, hormonal issues, and poor sleep may be an unaddressed emotional challenge that lies hidden deep within. Often, with the help of flower essences, the simple stresses of daily life can be lifted like a veil, allowing the sun to shine through and bringing with it the re-balance of body, mind, and spirit.

Accepting help from flower remedies doesn't mean that you don't address physical problems; but it does

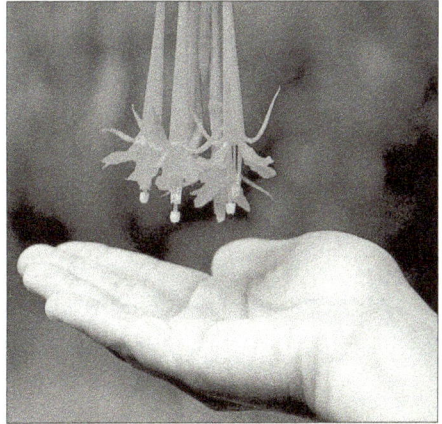

help you become aware of the emotional component of healing. Even during treatment for a physical ailment, we still need to have a positive outlook, which plays a vital role in the healing process. And that's why flower essences are so remarkable; they are powerful without being pushy. Their beauty lies in the fact that they gently restore harmony and balance without any side effects, so new problems don't arise while the existing ones are being treated.

HOMEOPATHY AND FLOWER ESSENCES

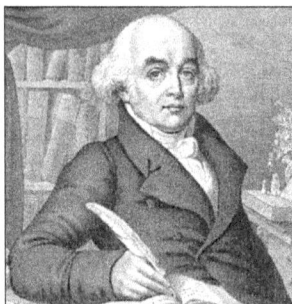

Dr. Samuel Hahnemann (1755-1843) was the father of homeopathy. He reasoned that there is a subtle energy force in the body, the vital force that responds to the remedies and enables the body to begin the healing process. Homeopathy preparations are serially diluted with shaking (succussing), thereby increasing the effect of the treatments, energizing and potenizing them with subtle energy. This dilution often continues until none of the original substance remains. Dr. Hahnemann observed from his experiments with Cinchona Bark, which is used as a treatment for malaria, that the effects from ingesting the bark were similar to the symptoms of malaria. He felt that the cure comes through similarity, using its properties to stimulate the body's own response to the disease. Through his continued experiments with other substances, he then concurred with the "Law of Similars;" widely known as "like cures like."

"The most beautiful thing we can experience is the mysterious."
–ALBERT EINSTEIN

The application of subtle energy is an aspect that is common to both homeopathy and flower essences; flower essences seem closest to the mother tincture of homeopathy. While they do have similarities, they also have differences.

When diagnosing using flower essences emotions and one's state of mind is primarily taken into account. Homeopathy does take the personality of the person into account, but it's mainly a complex science strongly orientation toward bodily suffering; a highly specific and symptom-orientated prescribing methodology.

THE BLOOM OF HEALING

Flower essences draw upon the "vibrational energy" of a plant's flower and, in most cases, are potentized naturally by the imprint of the medical dew of each flower. Medicinal dew is the pure dew on the plant or flower that becomes impregnated with the flower's healing power. It was the pioneers of flower essence therapy that discovered how to extract the healing power inherent in the flower's dew. Essences are made by floating the blossoms (picked at the optimal moment in the morning, while the dew is fresh) on the surface of a bowl of pure spring water, which is then placed in direct sunlight for several hours. For heartier plants and rocks, there is an alternative method that requires boiling. In both cases, sunlight aids in capturing the vibrational imprint of the flower or plant which is transferred to the water—that acts as a universal storage medium.

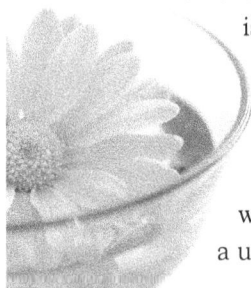

"I discovered the secret of the sea, in meditation upon the dewdrop."
–KAHLIL GIBRAN

On an early morning stroll through an open field, Dr. Bach observed the dew that lay heavy upon the land and flowers. It intuitively struck him that each dewdrop contained the property of the plant it rested on, and that the heat of the sun, acting through the fluid on the plant, drew out the plant's essence; the flower's innate healing power. He began to perfect a new method of extracting the dew, uncovering the energetic transference from plant to water. *In a paper written in the 1930s, Dr. Bach wrote about this process. In it he remarked:* ". . . the earth to nurture the plant, the air from which it feeds, the sun or fire to enable it to impart its power, and water to collect and be enriched with its beneficent magnetic healing."

EMPIRICAL RESEARCH

Flower essences were originally discovered through an intuitive observation and understanding of the plants from which the essences are derived. Since the qualities of certain flowers correspond to specific emotional patterns, these markers were, and continue to be, tested in clinical settings by health practitioners. Through scientific observation of their properties, the essences have been revised, expanded, or verified over the decades. This type of clinical study is called "empirical" research, and it is based on years of objective observation and experience. It is the primary method by which homeopathic remedies have been verified during the last two centuries. It is also the method that I use in my own flower essence trials, and the results are always remarkable, providing markers and insights that are sometimes subtle and often dramatic. Later on in the book, you will read about a number of research studies that have been carried out in several countries around the world.

"Men do not stumble over mountains, but over mole hills."
–CONFUCIUS

WHY THEY WORK

There is no simple answer to the question of why flower essences work. The many fine and subtle energy layers that surround us at any given moment can cause physical reactions as a result of the emotional and genetic baggage that we bring with us from birth, as well as the result of life experiences that unfold every moment. Because the body, mind, and spirit are interconnected, flower essences work on specific vibrational levels as holistic pathways that facilitate true balance, positive energy, and the restoration of our natural harmony. We often ask the question "why" when confronted with life's mysteries, and the best answer may simply be, "because."

An interesting aspect of flower essences is that when you take "the placebo effect" out of the equation with someone who is unconscious or comatose, infants, animals, and plants, the results are just as effective. Although understanding why you are taking the essences adds another healing component.

LIFE CYCLE OF FLOWER ESSENCES

I'm often asked, "Do I have to take flower essences forever? How long do they last?" Life is complicated and always changing. As the saying goes, "There is nothing permanent but change." We often heal in stages, with levels of clarity and insight appearing gradually—the clearing of lifelong issues rarely dissipates in an instant. Changes become stabilized when one's thoughts and actions continue to honor and support the lessons that we learn on life's path. For example: if we gather the strength and will to not overprotect a family member, over time, when another crisis arises, we may return to the same tendency. This is simply our natural inclination. Environment can be stronger than will, and emotional issues are not static, they change according to life's changes; as we release one issue a new one may arise. Flower essences address issues "in the moment," which, when used cumulatively, make up a lifelong journey! There will be long periods when essences are not required, when life is flowing just fine. And then, once again, a time may arise when either past or new issues present themselves. As part of the process of emotional growth, we address issues as they arise, cloud by cloud, in the ever-pristine blue sky of life.

Flower essences are very gentle, subtle, and don't linger in our system for long periods of time, which is why we can repeat them often in acute situations and why results are usually not spoken of in regards to a specific time frame. And then there are times when a single dose may provide the necessary insight or shed light on an emotional challenge—healing it once and for all!

"If you find yourself in a hole, the first thing to do is stop digging."
—WILL ROGERS

LAYERS OF HEALING

The healing process may take many months, especially when dealing with deeply ingrained anxieties that are caused by a domineering and inflexible personality, or when they are the lingering effects of childhood abuse or trauma. Ultimately, layers of repressed emotion or feelings begin to emerge, as well as sensations that may have been held deeply for years or even decades. It is important to take note of any negative feelings, as well as the positive ones, since this will

"Let us open our leaves like a flower, and be receptive."
—JOHN KEATS

provide valued insights into the application and use of each essence. With experience you can "read" these feelings and know when to stop, start, or introduce a new remedy.

ARE THE ESSENCES WORKING?

There are simple milestones that can be observed to determine if the essences are working. Often, people may simply feel renewed energy, a more positive attitude, or a greater ability to handle life's challenges—viewing them in a broader and more adaptable perspective. Whatever the reason you began taking flower essences in the first place may no longer seem as pressing or dominant. In more extreme cases, people generally do not feel so hopeless anymore, since there is often a growing realization that there *is* light at the end of the tunnel. With time, more insights can open one to emotional wounds that were long held, and when this is recognized they can finally begin to dissipate and heal.

> *"Nirvana is not the blowing out of the candle; it is the*
> *extinguishing of the flame because day is come."*
> —RABINDRANATH TAGORE

ARE FLOWER ESSENCES SAFE?

One of the wonderful aspects of flower essences is that they do not affect us biochemically the way traditional allopathic medicines do. Adding flower essence therapy to allopathic medicine never causes a risk of side effects or contra reactions. Both systems compliment each other wonderfully, since prescription medications often dull one's consciousness. Flower essences, on the other hand, create a positive awareness that clears one's consciousness, thereby mitigating many of the psychological effects attributed to allopathic medicine.

Over decades, hundreds of thousands of people have found

flower essences to be completely safe. If, for some reason, the essence isn't the one that corresponds to the emotional challenge one is taking the remedy for, it simply has no reaction at all. Working by resonance, an essence that does not relate to our challenge will simply not stimulate a response within us. You also don't have to be concerned about plant, flower, or tree allergies; each essence is the energetic imprint of the flower, harvested from its life force energy, so there is nothing inherent in it to cause an adverse reaction. What a wonderful gift!

If someone reports that they experience an adverse reaction to a remedy, it may be the mind playing a trick in order to deter the person from continuing their therapy. When a person truly understands that flower essences do not cause any negative physical or emotional reactions, and they allow themselves to courageously address latent and current life issues, they can begin to develop a positive spirit that fosters healing at the deepest level.

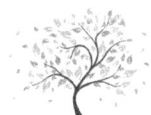

STARTING THE JOURNEY

"All glory comes from daring to begin." —WILLIAM SHAKESPEARE

Even though the many families of flower essences have the ability to address almost every emotional issue we face, we still have to factor in how much we desire to be well and whole. An example of this is the degree of urgency with which we seek harmony. A strong and sincere desire to be happy and free is essential. If we don't earnestly set out upon the journey, how can we possibly discover what we are looking for? Otherwise, it is like trying to climb a mountain but continually changing the path to the summit. At that rate, you will never reach the top.

It's good to ask oneself, "Am I ready to take the first step? Do I have the desire and courage to investigate and face the emotional issues that are arising right now, at this very moment?"

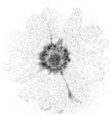

Chapter Two

THE DOCTRINE OF SIGNATURES

"In wilderness I sense the miracle of life, and behind it our scientific accomplishments fade to trivia."
—CHARLES A. LINDBERGH

"All things by immortal power, near and far. Hiddenly, to each other linked are, That thou canst not stir a flower, without troubling of a star."
–FRANCIS THOMPSON

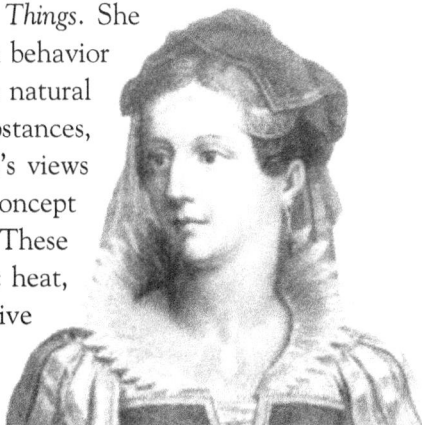

HERMETIC PRINCIPLE

In late medieval times, the world was filled with mystical images. "As above, so below" was a Hermetic principle which expressed the relationship between all that is large and infinite (macrocosm or universe-level), all the way down to the smallest and finite (microcosm, or sub-sub-atomic).

HILDEGARD VON BINGEN

In the twelfth century, Hildegard von Bingen (1098-1179) authored, *The Book of Subtleties of the Diverse Nature of Things.* She studied plants, trees, animals, birds, and human behavior and compiled her finding in this treatise on the natural world, the therapeutic powers of natural substances, and the doctrine of plant signatures. Hildegard's views stemmed from the Greek four-element theory, a concept which is based on fire, air, water, and earth. These elements correspond to four respective qualities: heat, dryness, moisture, and cold, and to four respective humors: choler (choleric), blood (sanguine), phlegm (phlegmatic), and black bile (melancholy).

"We cannot live only for ourselves. A thousand fibers connect us with our fellow men; and among those fibers, as sympathetic threads, our actions run as causes, and they come back to us as effects."
–HERMAN MELVILLE

"The soul is a breath of living spirit, that with excellent sensitivity, permeates the entire body to give it life. Just so, the breath of the air makes the earth fruitful. Thus the air is the soul of the earth, moistening it, greening it."
—HILDEGARD VON BINGEN

As with other medical practitioners of her time, Hildegard believed that illness stemmed from an imbalance in the humors and elements. She believed that prescribing the appropriate plant or natural substance would correct the imbalance and was the ideal way to restore health.

PARACELSUS

Almost four centuries later, Philippus Aureolus Theophrastus Bombastus von Hohenheim (1493-1541), the most famous advocate of signature plants (which takes into consideration the particular type of flower, where it grew, its color, scent, and its use for healing) arrived on the scene. This Swiss citizen, who later adopted the Latin name Paracelsus, published the literary work titled, *Doctrine of Signatures*.

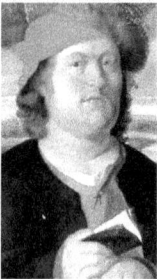

"Medicine is not only a science, it is also an art. It does not consist of compounding pills and plasters; it deals with the very processes of life, which must be understood before they may be guided. Once a disease has entered the body, all parts which are healthy must fight it: not one alone, but all, because a disease might mean their common death. Nature knows this, and Nature attacks the disease with whatever help she can muster."
—PARACELSUS

During the first half of the sixteenth century, Paracelsus travelled throughout Europe, Asia, and to Egypt, curing people with his natural remedies. He regularly experimented with new plants and always searched for more natural treatments and solutions. Paracelsus stated, "That which is looked upon by one generation as the apex of human knowledge is often considered an absurdity by the next, and that which is regarded as a superstition in one century may form the basis of science for the following one."

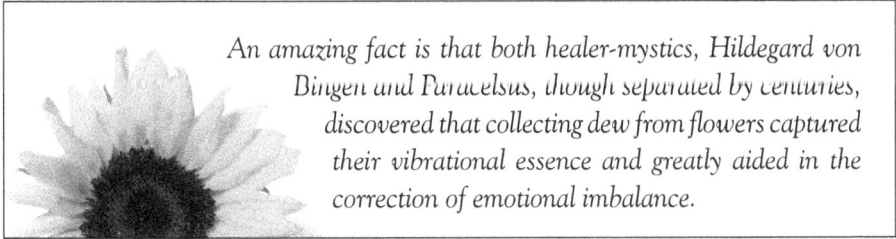

An amazing fact is that both healer-mystics, Hildegard von Dingen and Paracelsus, though separated by centuries, discovered that collecting dew from flowers captured their vibrational essence and greatly aided in the correction of emotional imbalance.

OTHER "DOCTRINE OF SIGNATURE" PROPONENTS

Giambattista della Porta was also a strong proponent of the theory of the doctrine of signatures. He was probably born in Naples shortly before the death of Paracelsus. His family surrounded themselves with distinguished men of the time and entertained prominent philosophers, mathematicians, poets, and musicians. He eventually wrote a book about human physiognomy, which incorporated the idea that the inner qualities and the healing power of herbs might also be revealed by external signs. This led to his famous work, *Phytognomonica*, which was first published in Naples in 1588. Both Paracelsus and Porta did not like the use of foreign drugs introduced to the body. They felt that the country where a disease arises can also host natural remedies as a means to overcome it. This idea is one which constantly recurs throughout the herbal remedy books during that time.

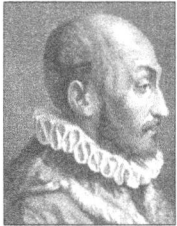

"You are not just a drop in the ocean. You are the mighty ocean in the drop."
—RUMI

Jakob Böhme (1575-1624) was a shoemaker from Görlitz, Germany, who claimed to have had a profound mystical vision as a young man, in which he saw the relationship between God and man revealed in all things. His writings and artwork were influenced and inspired by Paracelsus, the Kabbala, alchemy and the Hermetic tradition. He wrote, *Signatura Rerum* (1621), which was translated into English and named, *The Signature of All Things*. This spiritual doctrine was applied to the medicinal uses of plants.

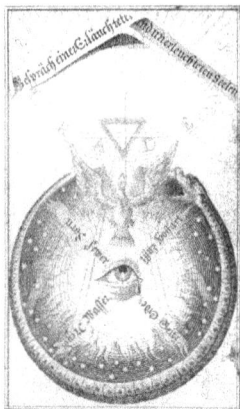

Böhme was a Theosophist, mystic, and artist. He created this image in 1682.

"Every flower is a soul blossoming in Nature."
—GERARD DE NERVAL

The idea that shapes of objects in nature have significance is a very ancient one and is not confined to Western thought. An example of this is the resemblance of the mandrake root to a human body, which led to its being ascribed great significance and special powers.

Additional examples of this early doctrine come from the seventeenth century botanist and herbalist William Coles (1626-1662), author of, *The Art of Simpling* and *Adam in Eden*. In his book, Coles stated that walnuts were good for curing head ailments because in his opinion, "They have the perfect signatures of the head." He wrote about *Hypericum* (Saint John's Wort): "The little holes whereof the leaves of Saint John's Wort are full, does resemble all the pores of the skin, and therefore it is profitable for all hurts and wounds that can happen thereunto."

Nicholas Culpeper (1616–1654), an early herbalist, described in his book, *Complete Herbal* the medical use of Foxglove—the botanical precursor to digitalis—for treating heart conditions. He also spoke about the doctrine of signatures as common knowledge and its influence in modern herbal lore.

Saint John's Wort

A well-known German poet and nature scientist, Johann Wolfgang von Goethe (1749-1832), took a holistic approach to

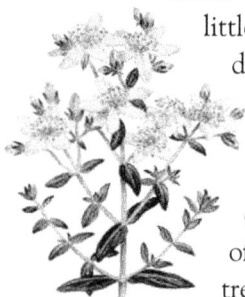

natural science. His soulful insight and connection to nature is reflected in his poem, *The Metamorphisis of Plants*:

"Sweetly concealed in the womb,
Where is made perfect the fruit.
Here doth Nature close the ring of her forces eternal;
Yet doth a new one, at once, cling to the one gone before,
So that the chain be prolonged forever through all generations."

Michel Foucault (1926-1984) was a French historian and philosopher who expressed a wider usage of the doctrine of signatures in his book, *The Order of Things*. In it he writes: "Up to the end of the sixteenth century, resemblance played a constructive role in the knowledge of Western culture. It was resemblance that largely guided interpretation of texts. It was the resemblance that organized the play of symbols, made possible knowledge of things visible and invisible, and controlled the art of representing them."

"Science is tending to show that life is harmony—a state of being in tune—and that disease is discord or a condition when a part of the whole is not vibrating in unison."
—Dr. Edward Bach

"The sun, with all those plants revolving around it and dependent upon it, can still ripen a bunch of grapes as if it had nothing else in the universe to do."
—Galileo Galilei

These theories and doctrines are found in mainstream medical texts far into the nineteenth century. It also played an influential role in the development of homeopathy, and in Dr. Edward Bach's discovery of the thirty-eight flower essences. The doctrine of signatures is not universally recognized by scientists since there is no definite evidence that plant signatures reveal medical uses of a respective plant. However, many of the flower essence pioneers found that there are often rational explanations for the apparent successes, especially in predicting the medical properties of certain plants. For example: a thorny plant may likely have immune-boosting compounds since it grows in an environment in which there are many external threats, and the plant needs a form of protection to survive.

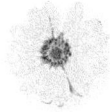

Chapter Three
THE SCIENTIFIC EXPLANATION

"It's likely that only vibrations of love and gratitude appear in nature, and observations of nature shows this to be true."
—MASARU-EMOTO

THE POWER OF POSITIVITY EXPERIMENTS

"Reality is the mirror of your thoughts. Choose well what you put in front of the mirror."
—REMEZ SASSON

t is well-known that a strong vibration influences a weaker one. A negative thought can often overpower a positive one, but the opposite is just as true. Since flower essences are living, positive vibrations, they work to initiate a condition that elevates us in a positive way. They act like an inspiring message or peaceful person who uplifts our spirit, then, like a mirror, we reflect the qualities we are exposed to.

Some interesting scientific research about the power of positivity has demonstrated that water has memory—the innate capacity to store information. A good example of this are experiments of Dr. Masaru-Emoto of Japan, who captured "expressions of water." Dr. Emoto discovered that crystals formed in frozen water reveal changes when specific, concentrated thoughts are directed toward them. He found that water from clear springs that had been exposed to loving words reveal brilliant, complex, and colorful snowflake patterns. In contrast, polluted water, or water exposed to negative thoughts form incomplete, asymmetrical patterns with

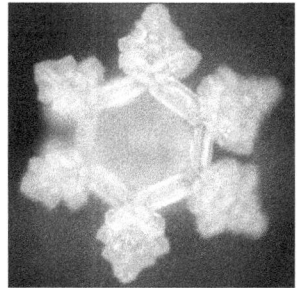

Emoto Water Crystal - Word "Love."

dull colors. The astounding implication of this research created a spectacular awareness of how we can positively impact not only the earth, but our personal health and well-being.

"You can do anything you think you can. This knowledge is literally the gift of the gods, for through it you can solve every human problem. It should make of you an incurable optimist. It is the open door."
—ROBERT COLLIER

THE RICE EXPERIMENT

Along with the water experiments, Dr. Emoto also asked people to try a rice experiment. You can try it, too:

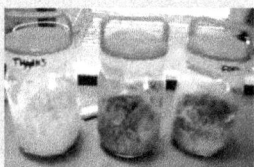

Three bottles of rice

Start with three jars with tight-fitting lids; make sure they are sterilized. Add one cup of cooked white rice to each jar. Label the first jar, "I love you, thank you." Label the second jar, "I hate you, you idiot." Don't label the third jar. Place the jars on a table about 18 inches apart and leave them there for one month. Each day state the positive message to the first jar, the negative message to the second jar, and simply ignore the third jar. In most cases, after one month, the "positive" jar grows a bright, colorful orange mold, while the "negative" jar is covered with a drab brown mold, and the "ignored" jar looks even worse!

This experiment shows that human consciousness can interact directly with the physical world. The results of the experiment support the understanding that life is interconnected, that we are affected by intentions in the environment around us, and we respond in entirely different ways. Positive and negative influences have the ability to *transform* our molecular structure. We absorb and store the energy and intentions from ourselves and others through thought and emotion. The interesting part of this experiment is that the "ignored" rice is the most affected. This shows us how important intention and awareness is.

VIBRATIONAL ENERGY IMPRINTING

Modern science and contemporary physics has demonstrated for nearly a century that matter and consciousness are intimately intertwined. To understand how flower essences work requires recognition that human beings are more than just a physical body, that they incorporate vital energy, intellectual understanding, and an innate spiritual consciousness.

> *"Nature, exerting an unwearied power, forms, opens,*
> *and gives scent to every flower."*
> —WILLIAM COWPER

Dr. Richard Gerber, in his book, *Vibrational Medicine*, provides a scientific and physiological description of how flower essences work. He says that when an essence is ingested or absorbed through the skin, it is initially assimilated into the blood stream, settling midway between the circulatory and nervous systems. The essence reaches the imbalanced parts of the body quickly and in a stable form. The quartz-like crystalline silica structures in the physical body, such as those in the bloodstream and the hair and nails, amplify and transmit the healing energies of flower essences to their appropriate and correct frequencies. He described the process as being similar to the way radio waves strike a crystal in a radio so that the crystal resonates with a high frequency, which absorbs and transforms them into audio frequencies that can be heard by the human ear.

"People like us, who believe in physics, know that the distinction between past, present, and future is only a stubbornly persistent illusion."
–ALBERT EINSTEIN

Since all of life is infused with an inborn intelligence, its natural inclination is toward harmony and balance. When this natural rhythm is out of sync, unease may occur, affecting both the body and mind. The therapeutic positive aspects of plants represent a form of "energetic essence therapy"; this "under-the-radar tool" promotes cellular health and optimum well-being. When flower essences are used for healing, it is always on a subtle level since they contain vibrational patterns of energy that interact and intersect with the patterns that help make up our physical and psychological being.

To understand the concept of multidimensional energy systems is to understand "matter as energy," which forms the basis of flower essence therapy. This realization, confirmed by Einstein, is presented in the theory of quantum physics—it is the understanding that matter and energy are only *apparently* separate expressions in the totality of existence.

Einstein's illumined understanding of the universe is well worth noting, he says:

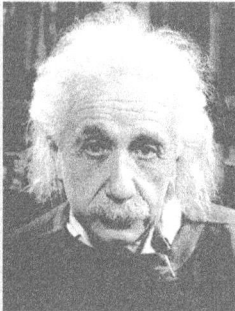

Albert Einstein

"A human being is a part of a whole, called by us—universe—a part limited in time and space. A person experiences themselves, their thoughts and feelings as something separated from the rest . . . a kind of optical delusion of consciousness. This delusion is a kind of prison for us, restricting us to our personal desires and to affection for a few persons nearest to us. Our task must be to free ourselves from this prison by widening our circle of compassion to embrace all living creatures and the whole of nature in its beauty."

The vibrational rate of universal energy determines its manifestation within the world of matter: physical matter vibrates at lower frequencies; subtle or spiritual matter vibrates at higher frequencies.

Therefore, flower essences don't attack disease but, in simple terms, restore healthy resonating frequencies.

Utilizing principals that are similar to homeopathy, flower essences have the power to imprint the vibrational character within a particular plant's core. *The concept was beautifully expressed by Dr. Edward Bach this way:*

> "The action of flower essences raises the vibration of being . . . they cure by flooding the body with the beautiful vibrations of the highest nature in whose presence there is the opportunity for disease to melt away like snow in sunshine."

Vibrational or energetic essence therapy operates similarly to the way a tuning fork does. It you have two tuning forks next to each other, by striking one, you make the other vibrate at the same frequency. When we use flower essences to restore balance, the flowers' vibration triggers positive changes in our emotional energy.

It may be that the very cures of our modern age have always been held within the seed of this ancient truth: that energetic healing is and has always been *present* in nature. Actually, we are only just rediscovering this complementary healing system, which has reemerged in the last hundred years.

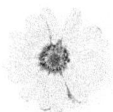

Chapter Four

USING FLOWER ESSENCES

*"Can we conceive what humanity would be
if it did not know flowers?"*
—MAURICE MAETERLINCK

THE SELECTION JOURNEY

Selecting the right flower essences is often part of a process of inner growth and awareness. Through quiet reflection, meditation, self-observation, and consultation, we all have the ability to become aware of issues that need resolution; issues related to our work, relationships, or inner conflicts. You can start the journey by using the checklists and guides at the end of this chapter, to identify the issues that need to be addressed. Then you can begin to review and study the flower essence selection guide (page 106), purchase flower essence books, or work with any of the online resources.

Selecting the right essence(s), can paradoxically be both simple and complex. There are a number of essences that work on stress, but they often have subtle differences. Understanding and intuiting which essence or combination of essences will work best for your condition may take some experimentation. Examples of subtle differences from the Bach family are:

- *Holly* is for an outward explosive anger; *Willow* is for a more inward, smoldering anger.
- *Olive* is for extreme mental or physical overwork; *Hornbeam*

is for a sense of exhaustion at the very thought of work.

- *Chicory* is for possessiveness of family or loved ones; *Red Chestnut* is for fearfulness and worry about those loved ones.
- *Water Violet* is a reluctance to show feelings from a sense of pride; *Agrimony* pretends everything is fine and puts on a happy facade.
- *Oak* is for people who overwork, never giving themselves a break; *Elm* is for responsible people who temporarily feel overwhelmed.

FLOWER ESSENCES FOR MEDITATION & FOCUS

If you find your mind unable to focus, especially when trying to choose an essence, your mental energy may be dissipated. Focusing the mind is a meditation exercise just like any physical exercise and improves with practice. You can use it for clarity during the selection process. A good time to use the flower essences are prior to meditation.

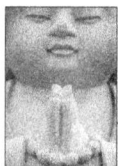

Flower Essence Meditation

Find a quiet place and sit in a comfortable position. Place two drops of an essence on your tongue or a dab of cream on your forehead. [Suggestions: *Solomon's Seal*, *Lotus*, or *White Chestnut*]. Whatever approach you use for meditation, simply let your mind be a passive observer and the "flower essence" your partner in calming your mind and heart. If a strong emotion or feeling arises don't resist it, observe it nonreactively and stay rooted as the observer. You can also watch your breathing to help keep your focus and attention. The main object is not to stop thoughts—since they arise naturally—but to not get caught up in them. If you discover that you are engaging a passing thought, bring your mind back to observing your breath. You don't need to employ a formal sitting meditation to receive the therapeutic benefits of a calm and clear mind. You can attune yourself to stillness and universal consciousness anytime, anywhere. You are never away from it, even in the midst of traffic—and it's especially useful during those times!

"Life is a train of moods like a string of beads; and as we pass through them they prove to be many colored lenses, which paint the world their own hue, and each shows us only what lies in its own focus."
—Ralph Waldo Emerson

DISCOVERING EMOTIONS & STATES OF MIND

Have you noticed that there are some days when you just feel sad for no particular reason? From past experience you know this feeling will pass. It's the same with the feelings of extreme surprise or extreme fear. They bring us right into the moment and all life's nonessentials fade into the background. If we don't overreact by putting up walls or barriers to these emotions, they will go their own way without adding any ripples, like a cloud flitting across the blue sky. It is when the emotion or states of mind linger that we get caught up in them, and through this emotional identification we create limiting beliefs about ourselves and others. If we can recognize a particular emotion as it arises, we can deal with it in real time before it spirals out of control.

"The greatest discovery of any generation is that a human being can alter his life by altering his attitude."
—William James

But not all emotions are bad, since they represent one of the fundamental traits that make us human. Emotions often color people's lives and give them great depth and richness. For many people, strong emotions are linked to creativity and expression. Great art, music, and literature—at least on a fundamental level—creates a special emotional connection between the artist or musician and the way the piece is perceived by the audience.

A state of mind is an attitude, which is often assumed to be the simplest component of thought. This implies that a person can have different mental postures toward an intention, as in: believing, desiring, clinging, craving, etc. In the world of flower essences, you need to explore both emotions and states of mind in order to begin the healing journey using this complementary therapy.

A good exercise to discover your emotions and states of mind are to pose a few questions to yourself:

How does allowing life to happen, without reacting, make me feel?

How does resisting what *is* happening make feel?
Am I feeling in harmony or am I stressed?
How does stress affect my ability to respond to people and events?

Without even answering these questions, but by simply mulling them, you can feel what stirs within you, what makes you feel good, and what makes you feel uncomfortable. It's an inner investigation.

"Sometimes questions are more important than answers."
–NANCY WILLARD

SEVEN BACH EMOTIONAL GROUPS

Dr. Edward Bach separated his remedies into seven emotional groups. Like the exercise above we can go through the list and ask questions to figure out which emotional group we are experiencing at any time, such as:

1. Am I fearful? What kind of fear is it?
2. Do I feel uncertain? What uncertainty is happening right now?

Here are seven groups categorized by Dr. Bach; the detailed list of which essences belong to each category are listed on page 128:

1. Fear
2. Uncertainty
3. Insufficient interest in present circumstances
4. Loneliness
5. Oversensitivity to influences and ideas
6. Despondency or despair
7. Overcare for welfare of others

REASONS TO CHOOSE TREATMENT

There are certain key categories that affect our lives, and when there is imbalance in any of these areas, the challenges may become more layered and complex. Can you recognize any of them in yourself?

*"Relaxation means releasing all concern and tension and letting
the natural order of life flow through one's being."*
—DONALD CURTIS

RELAXATION

Stress is experienced in epidemic proportions these days. It is well-known that up to 85% of lifestyle problems have their root in stress. We are often deep in the throngs of stress before we even recognize that we have succumbed to its grip. One of the main properties inherent in flower essences is the ability to act as powerful stress-releasers in a wide variety of situations.

"Energy and persistence conquer all things."
—BENJAMIN FRANKLIN

VITAL ENERGY

Many emotional and psychological issues, which tax our energy, often grow from a small stream into a river of various debilitating conditions. Allopathic treatments like chemotherapy and strong drug regimes cause a variety of side-effects, especially in depleting energy.

*"You will never be happier than you expect.
To change your happiness, change your expectation."*
—BETTE DAVIS

HAPPINESS AND CONTENTMENT

We are naturally wired to desire to be happy, just as a bee is naturally programmed to find nectar. We all seek happiness in everything we do, even in seemingly negative behaviors. However, happiness is regularly being challenged by so many factors: grief, distress, and obsession, to name just a few. Flower essences, when properly used, have the unique ability to draw upon one's innate positive energy and help bring us back to peace, healing, and balance.

"In joy or sadness, flowers are our constant friends."
—KOZUKO OKAKURA

MOODS

The variety of moods that make us sad, angry, worried, etc., are a powerful precursor that go on to create other, more prominent problems and general discontent. Remaining balanced and free from the influence of our moods will help bring us back into harmony and freedom. Flower essences work especially well in balancing moods.

"People do change, and change comes like a little wind that ruffles the curtains at dawn, and it comes like the stealthy perfume of wildflowers hidden in the grass."
—JOHN STEINBECK

CHANGE

Change is a big factor, because life is always changing. Some people are challenged by change more than others. In fact, it may be their main issue. If we cannot, like the willow tree, bend in the wind, rigidity may snap us in half. Working through and accepting change can bring great relief. On the other hand, some people are addicted to change and cannot relax without becoming bored, which can be just as paralyzing.

"To conquer fear is the beginning of wisdom."
—BERTRAND RUSSELL

FEAR

There are many aspects to fear that need to be addressed; we often find it easier to hide from them. Fear comes in the form of a myriad of known things, as well as the illusive and shadowy fear of the unknown. When fear is no longer a factor, one is truly free.

"Let go of the life we have planned;
accept the life that is waiting for us."
—JOSEPH CAMPBELL

LETTING GO

Our nature is to attach ourselves to our family, our possessions, our thoughts, and our opinions. In truth, it is only when we let go that we can truly begin to hold on to what we have. This is one of life's great paradoxes.

"Truth is not far away; it is ever present. It is not something to be attained,
since not one of your steps leads away from it."
—DOGEN

SPIRITUAL AWARENESS

Without integrating spiritual awareness into our consciousness, we often find ourselves disconnected. Flower essences help to promote peace and harmony in all aspects of our life, with an integrative connection with everything and everyone we come in contact with.

THE LAYERS OF HUMAN EMOTION

The classic psychological reference to human emotions is many layers deep and can be classified as primary, secondary, and tertiary. The primary emotions are love, joy, surprise, anger, sadness, and fear. To begin a flower essence treatment program, it is important to pinpoint the emotions that are challenging us at the moment. Once we target them we can begin to address them.

Love: Love often develops from a feeling of profound oneness. It can be platonic, romantic, religious, or familial, and there are certain nuances to love in regards to bonding, friendship, unselfishness, and charity.

Joy: Joy or happiness has endless shades of enjoyment, satisfaction, and pleasure. There is a sense of harmony, well-being, inner peace, love, safety, and contentment that is attached to this emotion. But there can also be a negative component when surrounded with past feelings and experiences. We may cling to a former joyful memory and not be able to move forward. The layers are endless.

Surprise: Surprise means experiencing an unexpected result. Emotions that emanate from surprise are astonishment and amazement. It may also relate to the inability to accept change, being surprised by expectations gone awry.

Anger: Anger may be evoked due to many factors: injustice, conflict, humiliation, negligence, or betrayal. Anger can also be a cause of hidden trauma—a response to a past, unpleasant event. On a less negative note, it may also arise when we feel at conflict or at odds with strong idealistic feelings. The magnitude of anger and its underlying source is what one needs to perceive to truly understand it.

Sadness: Sadness is often related to feelings of loss and difficulties. When not addressed and left to fester, it can lead to despondency and depression.

Fear: Fear is a response to some danger that is about to happen. It is nature's survival mechanism that reacts to a negative stimulus. At times it is only a mild caution, or it can become extreme and irrational.

PRIMARY, SECONDARY, AND TERTIARY EMOTIONS

Use this chart to identify emotions or states of mind. Note which Tertiary emotion(s) relate to you at this moment.

PRIMARY	SECONDARY	TERTIARY
LOVE	Affection	Adoration, fondness, attraction, caring, tenderness, compassion, sentimentality, devotion, good will, kindness
	Lust	Arousal, desire, passion, infatuation, longing, sensuality, urge
	Longing	Anxiousness, craving, wishfulness, yearning
JOY	Cheerfulness	Amusement, bliss, glee, jolliness, joy, delight, enjoyment, gladness, happiness, satisfaction, ecstasy, euphoria, optimism
	Zest	Enthusiasm, zeal, excitement, exhilaration, passion, ecstasy
	Contentment	Pleasure, serenity, peace, fulfillment, satisfaction
	Pride	Conceit, disdain, vanity, egoism, pretension
	Optimism	Eagerness, hope, certainty, easiness, calmness
	Relief	Alleviation, balm, comfort, contentment
SURPRISE	Amazement	Astonishment, shake-up, aghast, wonderment
ANGER	Irritation	Aggravation, agitation, annoyance, grumpiness, discomfort, tension, irritability, anger, stress
	Exasperation	Frustration, annoyance, displeasure, resentment
	Rage	Outrage, fury, hostility, bitterness, hate, spite, vengefulness
	Disgust	Revulsion, contempt, loathing, displeasure
	Envy	Jealousy, malice, rivalry, spite, prejudice, upset, craving
	Injustice	Botheration, exasperation, frustration
SADNESS	Suffering	Hurt, anguish, pain, difficulty, misfortune, ordeal
	Sadness	Depression, despair, hopelessness, gloom, unhappiness, grief, sorrow, misery, melancholy, blues, heartbreak
	Disappointment	Dismay, discouragement, displeasure, despondency, frustration
	Shame	Regret, remorse, guilt, humiliation, confusion, debasement
	Neglect	Alienation, isolation, loneliness, rejection, homesickness, defeat, insecurity, embarrassment, slovenliness
	Sympathy	Pity, empathy, understanding, compassion
FEAR	Horror	Shock, fear, fright, terror, panic, hysteria, dread, aversion
	Nervousness	Anxiety, tenseness, uneasiness, apprehension, worry, distress, tension, fright, timidity, jitters

Flower Essence Awareness Quiz

Circle a number from 0—10.
0 doesn't apply at all • 5 leaning in that direction • 10 completely agree.

Below are some sample statements, write your own statements and keep them in a notebook. While using the flower essence combinations you have chosen for yourself, you can check back to see if specific emotional issues have changed or have stayed the same.

Sample Statements

1. I feel completely exhausted; I can't accomplish what I set out to do.
   0   1   2   3   4   5   6   7   8   9   10

2. I am feeling restless and can't sit still.
   0   1   2   3   4   5   6   7   8   9   10

3. I am constantly worried about my family.
   0   1   2   3   4   5   6   7   8   9   10

4. I feel very distracted, scattered, and not present.
   0   1   2   3   4   5   6   7   8   9   10

5. I am having difficultly letting go of the past to begin something new.
   0   1   2   3   4   5   6   7   8   9   10

6. My life is filled with too many overwhelming responsibilities right now.
   0   1   2   3   4   5   6   7   8   9   10

7. I feel deeply discouraged and despondent, whatever happens affects me.
   0   1   2   3   4   5   6   7   8   9   10

8. I am feeling gloomy and depressed for no real reason.
   0   1   2   3   4   5   6   7   8   9   10

9. I have no patience.
   0   1   2   3   4   5   6   7   8   9   10

10. I feel unappreciated for all the work I do for others.
   0   1   2   3   4   5   6   7   8   9   10

> *"Beneath words and logic are emotional connections that largely direct how we use our words and logic."*
> —JANE ROBERTS

Checklist

"Our emotional symptoms are precious sources of life and individuality."
–THOMAS MORE

This is a helpful exercise for uncovering emotional blocks that may be in your life. It is a good place to start because it can reveal issues that may have been pushed into the background.

This checklist is a subtle word association exercise. Try not to think too much when answering. Simply react. Let the unconscious mind respond to these questions. If a response doesn't apply, leave it blank. There are degrees to which any of these emotions may apply, but try to focus on the ones that are most pressing and need to be addressed. This exercise can help point you toward selecting the right remedy. You will still need to research the various flower essences to determine which ones would best heal the revealed challenges.

Sometimes an issue may be apparent, but oftentimes it will take the unraveling of layers of emotional baggage before a greater understanding is achieved.

Note: Copy this page or use a separate piece of paper to record your responses, so you can come back to this checklist whenever you need to.

ABOUT FEELINGS
Check the feelings you are experiencing now.

(_) rejection	(_) confusion
(_) doubt	(_) betrayal
(_) regret	(_) anger
(_) depressed	(_) hatred
(_) abandonment	(_) vengefulness
(_) weakness	(_) grief
(_) exhaustion	(_) pride
(_) injustice	(_) frustration

Other:

ABOUT EXPECTATIONS
Check your heightened expectations of the following:

(__) unrealistic expectations of yourself
(__) expectations of children
(__) expectations of spouse or loved one
(__) expectations of peers, associates or clients (work related)
(__) expectations of friends and acquaintances
(__) expectations of career or personal interests
Other:

ABOUT RELATIONSHIPS
Check if you experience fear of or guilt associated with any the following:

(__) fear of anger   (__) guilt associated with anger
(__) fear of feelings   (__) guilt associated with feelings
(__) fear of emotions   (__) guilt associated with no emotions
(__) fear of parents   (__) guilt associated with parents
(__) fear of children   (__) guilt associated with children
(__) fear of intimacy   (__) guilt associated with intimacy
(__) fear of God   (__) guilt associated with religion
(__) fear of spouse   (__) guilt associated with spouse or family
(__) fear of social engagement   (__) guilt associated with not socializing
(__) fear of peer pressure   (__) guilt associated with peers or clients
(__) fear of financial security   (__) guilt of excessive financial situation
(__) fear of taking risks   (__) guilt of irresponsible risk-taking
(__) fear of being deceived   (__) guilt of one's own deception
(__) fear of being manipulated   (__) guilt of one's own manipulation
(__) fear of abuse   (__) guilt of victimization or abuse
(__) fear of violence   (__) guilt of violence
(__) fear of betrayal   (__) guilt of betraying others
Other:

DESIRES

Check which desires you are aspiring for at the moment.

(__) acceptance
(__) success (this is a relative term; everyone's definition of success
    is their own, but see if this stirs a particular emotion)
(__) freedom
(__) love
(__) control
(__) intimacy
(__) security
(__) solitude
Other:

"Painful as it may be, a significant emotional event can be the catalyst for choosing a direction that serves us—and those around us—more effectively.

Look for the learning."
–LOUISA MAY ALCOTT

PERSONAL STORY

Write down your personal story. This can be a few paragraphs or simply bits of various thoughts. The story should include what is affecting you and the emotions that surround the issue(s) you are facing at this time. It should also provide an overview of your personality, temperament, and immediate attitudes. The act of putting words to paper is often therapeutic. Once the words are in front of you, it will be easier to sort through your feelings.

> *"Men are disturbed not by things,*
> *but by the view which they take of them."*
> —EPICTETUS

CREATING A FLOWER ESSENCE JOURNAL

Another way to select and use flower essences is by keeping a journal of your daily thoughts, dreams, and significant feelings. This is a helpful way to monitor any changes you may be experiencing. Since flower essences guide and heal in a gentle and subtle way, you may not easily notice shifts in patterns that have changed during short periods of time until you actually go back and review your journal. With new vibrational patterns of energy in your life, you may find it easier to discover the inner tools that allow you to become the creative designer of your life.

1. In a bound journal, notebook, or even on a computer, give yourself ten to twenty minutes each day to write.

2. Record emotions you feel at the time you are writing.

3. Don't plan what you are going to write, just write! Write down everything that comes into your mind without stopping or editing; let it be a stream of consciousness. The words you write may be funny, sad, angry, silly, or happy. Any emotions that come out are fine. The positive expressions are as important as the negative one's, since they help you to feel grateful for the good things that you have in your life.

4. You can also frame the words as a letter to someone.

5. Try to write everyday. You don't need to share your journal with anyone. These are your words and they hold your private thoughts. You need to be completely honest and express yourself without any inhibitions, fear, or concern.

6. After a few weeks of writing, look back at what you have written. See what things you have accomplished, what stressor has resolved itself and what stressor hasn't. Use your journal as a tool to explore issues like self-esteem and self-confidence.

7. You can even create an online journal. Use this link: *www.my-diary.org*

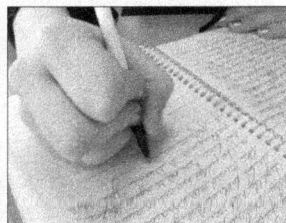

Enjoy the Journey!

FINDING JUST THE RIGHT ESSENCE

Once you establish what your specific challenges are you will need to discover just the right essence, or combination of essences, that are best suited for your situation. Unless you are a flower essence practitioner familiar with properties inherent in hundreds of essences, you will need to do some research. The resources at the end the book can provide an excellent start; online resources are also available. You can even make a set of flash cards (see page 126).

"All learning has an emotional base."
*–*Plato

The benefits of using a flower essence practitioner are many, especially since it allows you to take full advantage of their expertise. Essence combinations may actually cost less *with* a consultation as opposed to purchasing the many bottles you'll need. However, this should not deter you from your own research into flower essences; it is an exciting and fulfilling journey of discovery.

REMEMBERING TRIGGERS

A good way to start learning about the properties in flower essences is to associate a character from a novel, a specific person you know who resembles the property of an essence, or even a song lyric.

Examples of this are:
  Mimulus: "Little Miss Muffet" who was afraid of a spider.
  Cherry Plum: the song, "I think I'm going out of my head."
  Little Flannel Flower: the famous quote by Nadine Stair, "If
      I had my life to live over I'd pick more daises."
  Morning Glory: Rip Van Winkle who slept for twenty years.
  Honeysuckle: the story of the boy who wouldn't grow up,
      Peter Pan.

Another good way to remember specific essences is to become an observer of people. Watch and listen; see how people react to their environment. As you notice what unfolds in front of you try to discover a flower essence that might benefit the person in that moment.

When determining a pressing emotional issue or state of mind that needs rebalancing, it is also important to consider the whole person, including personality and lifestyle.

An example of this is five women giving birth in the same clinic:
- *Red Grevillea* is overly-possessive, not letting her husband leave her side.
- *Agrimony* is terrified, but no one would know—she is smiling and stoic.
- *Elm*, a highly responsible executive, is having a temporary but nagging doubt that she doesn't have the strength to go through with it.
- *Black-Eyed Susan* walks nervously up and down the hall, even though the doctor asks her to rest.
- *Beech* is highly critical and judgemental of the very staff helping to make this the most wonderful day of her life.

While addressing personalities, there may be a few things the previously mentioned women all have in common: exhaustion, self-image, hormonal mood swings, and a sense of apprehension, especially if it is their first child.

A few examples of common essences for pregnancy and birth:
- *Alpine Lily* helps reproductive organs experience conception and pregnancy as positive states.
- *Mariposa Lily* promotes warmth and nurturing; mother-child bonding.
- *Olive* for extreme exhaustion.
- *Bottlebrush* is a general essence for pregnancy; life changes.
- *Macrocarpa* helps revitalize the body after the trials of labor.

There are even essences for the newborn baby:
- *Star of Bethlehem* for the shock and trauma of birth; helps soothe and comfort.
- *Chamomile* especially works well to harmonize babies for greater emotional peace, serenity, and equanimity. What a wonderful way to come into the world!

An important discovery was made by Dr. Bach when, quite reluctantly, he was asked to attend a formal dinner. To pass the time, he began to observe the people around him. It dawned on him, as a flash of intuition, that humanity consisted of a number of "groups." He noticed that every individual in the large hall belonged to one group or another. Dr. Bach observed how they ate their food, how they smiled and moved their hands and heads, the attitudes of their bodies, the expressions on their faces and the tones of their voices. He saw that the resemblance between certain people were so close that they seem to belong to the same family. By the time the dinner was over, he had worked out twelve specific types of groups. What Dr. Bach identified were groups of personality traits, archetypal patterns of behavior.

FLOWER ESSENCE DOSAGE

The most common way to administer up to seven different flower essences is to make a combination bottle and add a few drops of preservation. Fill a mixing bottle with noncarbonated spring or purified water, and a small amount of brandy or apple cider. For alcohol sensitive people you can use vegetable glycerin or an extract of red shiso, purple mint; often used in macrobiotic cooking.

Flower essences may also be added to bath water, lotions, creams, oils, a baby's bottle, or a pet's water supply. The number of drops used in each flower essence family varies and ranges between two to eight drops. There are a number of already combined essences like *Rescue Remedy*®, which counts as only one essence.

You can use a single essence or a combination in the same way. They are generally taken orally by putting two to four drops directly under the tongue or by adding the drops to juice or water. More is not better since taking extra drops are not necessary. In the case of acute situations, you may increase the effect of an essence by taking it more frequently. For instance, during a time of great anxiety, essences may be taken up to five minutes apart until you begin to feel relief. Bedtime and mornings are especially effective dosage times. Flower essence tinctures should always be stored out of direct sunlight and away from heat and humidity. (See complete dosage details on page 134-135).

Allow your inner voice to speak to you about the length of time to continue taking a particular essence. Generally, flower essence practitioners recommend taking an essence or combination for a least three to four weeks. After the month, you can re-evaluate to see if you feel the need to continue or change the essence(s). Oftentimes, forgetting to take your remedies may indicate that another essence is in order, or that a separate issue has arisen. Looking at it in another way, if you are feeling balanced and happy, you may have resolved the issue you began treatment for in the first place.

"The best thing about the future is that it comes one day at a time."
—ABRAHAM LINCOLN

FLOWER ESSENCE COMBINING

During my many years of practice, I have found that most people require more than one essence. An issue is not always singular in nature, but often comprised of a complex rainbow of emotional, personality, and psychological overlays. In rare cases, only one essence is needed, and sometimes just a few doses may do the trick. Combining the appropriate essences can bring balance and fullness to the outcome. I often start with the Bach family as a foundation then choose from other groups of flower essences (up to seven or eight). A study of flower essences has shown that there are millions of possible combinations, making flower essences a complete and synergistic healing approach.

"Emotion always has its roots in the unconscious and manifests itself in the body."
–IRENE CLAREMONT DE CASTILLEJO

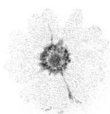

Chapter Five

CHILDREN AND ANIMALS

"Every child is born a naturalist. His eyes are, by nature, open to the glories of the stars, the beauty of the flowers, and the mystery of life."
—R. SEARCH

CHILDREN

Children have a special affinity to the gentle healing properties found in flowers. They respond quickly to flower essences because they are extremely sensitive beings, and their tiny bodies and minds resonate with positive energy. Flower essences can help a fussy baby or child become peaceful, the shy and fearful child find courage, and the impatient and angry child find peace.

The therapeutic properties of flower essences work to calm children, especially those overstimulated by the fast-paced world they find themselves in. The safe, natural aspects of this therapy mean that parents do not need to worry about any adverse side effects.

Parents whose children have used flower essences from babyhood to the teen years often report back that they notice a tremendous difference between their children and others that were not given this advantage. The flower essence children often develop an expanded range of emotional expressiveness and generally exhibit greater courage when moving forward in the world. I can attest to this in watching my own flower essence daughter blossom through life.

"In the long history of humankind (and animal kind, too) those who learned to collaborate and improvise most effectively have prevailed."
–CHARLES DARWIN

Since babies and children are not able to clearly verbalize their needs or problems, it is helpful to develop the art of listening and observation in order to determine emotional clues. For children over two years old, one of the best methods to decipher specific issues is through art, since their inner emotions are easily expressed through this creative outlet.

"Drawing is like making an expressive gesture
with the advantage of permanence."
—Henri Matisse

A wonderful example of flower essences for children is the story of Beth Beasley. She was a dedicated mother of an autistic child, Jarrett, who was on twenty-two medicines a day, many of which were antidepressants. She decided to incorporate flower essences into his daily routine and change them according to his needs each day. The end result was that her son began to show empathy and affection and a new inclination to listen and follow directions. Jarrett's doctors were amazed that this was the same little boy who first came to them, especially when he told his therapist, "Mommy made me better with the flowers from God." (See page 129 for autism drop combination.)

Administering to children is easily accomplished using drops in water, creams, and misters. Creams are helpful for babies and very young children since they can be massaged onto the skin, and light massage is very soothing to them. I also recommend playing classical or relaxing music while you do this. The positive, calming vibration of music adds to the healing effect. For older children and teens, misters are ideal, you can mist their rooms, it generally works like a charm.

Since children are highly sensitive beings, they quickly absorb and react to the environment in which they are placed. Flower essences open them to this resonant, positive energy, which helps them navigate through their own set of unique challenges. This, in turn, gives them a solid emotional foundation that will serve them for the rest of their lives.

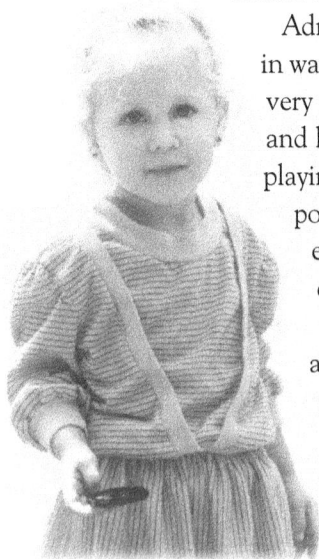

"A dog wags its tail with its heart."
—Martin Buxbaum

ANIMAL CHALLENGES

Because most animals live in a state of innate harmony with their surroundings, they don't become as imbalanced as humans do. However, animals have emotions, attitudes, and distinct personalities. One can observe and learn how to distinguish between their normal behavior and behavior that is out of sync for them. Also, pets sometimes react to the emotions of the people they are devoted to. Animals respond quickly and positively to flower essences; they are safe and self-correcting, and the placebo effect is taken out of the equation.

"An animal's eyes have the power to speak a great language."
—Martin Buber

A good way to administer to animals is through the use of a spray bottle. You can spray the animal's living space, put it in their bath water, in their drinking bowl, or simply spray it on your hands and massage it into their skin. There are a number of emotional and psychological issues in which flower essences can benefit animals. Several of them include: abuse, neglect or abandonment, fear of loud noises (like thunder), listlessness, anxiety, hyperactivity, aggressiveness, jealousy, or changes in their environment.

An interesting example was when we used flower essences on our pet bird, Mimi, a female cockatiel that was very attached to my husband. We decided to add a male bird to our household to give Mimi some companionship. It completely backfired; Mimi became so jealous that she began attacking Lee Lee, the new bird, to the extent that we were afraid for his life. So, we had a battle on our hands. I immediately added *Holly* (for jealousy) to Mimi's water bottle. Within a few days it all turned around. Mimi stopped bothering the new bird, and although they never formed a close attachment, they did learn to live in peace with each other.

You may want to try flower essences before you go on vacation or when there is a major change in your pet's life.

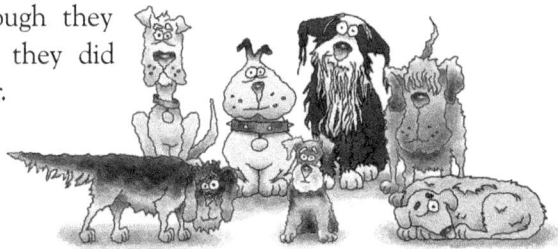

ESSENCES FOR CHILDREN AND ANIMALS

Here are a few examples of flower essences' healing abilities:

CHILDREN
For adoption
Mariposa Lily: This is especially helpful to bring freedom and healing from separation and alienation. Helps a child become more receptive to love.
Boronia: Helps with detachment issues; good for children who have a difficult time with new relationships.

For fearful and shy children
Mimulus: For specific fears and also for shyness; teaches courage and strength.
Bush Fuchsia: Courage and clarity in interacting with others.

For manipulation:
Chicory: Helps children through periods of selfishness, especially in the manipulation of parents, siblings, and friends.

For not learning from past mistakes:
Chestnut Bud: Helps children who make the same mistake over and over again. Also good for children who have difficulty in learning.
Black Spruce: Helps those with a tendency to forget information learned from past experiences. Good for a child out of touch with his or her inner wisdom.

ANIMALS
For hyperactivity:
Impatiens: For the "type A" animal filled with nervous energy.
Solomon's Seal: Helps an overactive animal to relax.

For abandonment or abuse:
Holly: To counterbalance jealousy, envy, suspicion, and anger.

For trauma:
Ashoka Flower: For deep-seated disharmony from any trauma.
Rock Rose: For terror and panic after an accident or terrifying event.

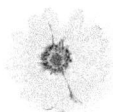

Chapter Six
WORLDWIDE FLOWER ESSENCE FAMILIES

"I believe a leaf of grass is no less than the journey-work of the stars."
—WALT WHITMAN

FLOWER ESSENCE PIONEERS AND A SELECTION OF ESSENCES

In the previous chapters, we have explored the ways to use flower essences to heal oneself. Our innate connection with nature spans cultures: from the Aboriginal tribes of Australia to the early settlers of the African plains; from the ancient Egyptians who perfected the art of aromatherapy to the thriving Ayurvedic culture in India; from early natural healing practices throughout Asia and South America to the North American Native Peoples' integration of nature and spirit.

In Chapter Two, we also looked at the historical background and early folklore of flower essences, which dates back to medieval times, documenting the understanding of plants and flowers core healing properties transferred to its dew.

This discovery seemed to have been lost—or simply receded into the background—until Dr. Edward Bach (1886-1936) brought it back from the brink. This was followed by a host of healers from around the world who pioneered, and continue to discover, the art of healing with flower essences. In many of these

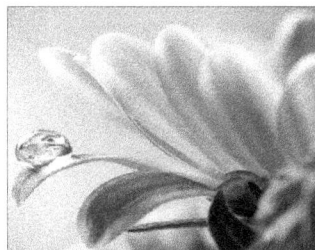

practices initially inspired by Dr. Bach, they often use his water formula and boiling method for extracting the healing properties of the flowers' subtle yet powerful therapeutic medicinal dew.

In his first book on flower essences, *Heal Thyself*, Dr. Bach wrote: "And so come out, my brothers and sisters, into the glorious sunshine of the knowledge of your Divinity, and earnestly and steadfastly set to work to join in the grand Design of being happy and communicating happiness . . ."

In this chapter, we explore flower essence pioneers, their colorful history, as well as highlight a selection of their remedies: the type of flower or plant it is, its family genesis, where it grows, and their unique healing characteristics. These are but a few of the characters in the epic novel we call, *Flower Essences*. It is my hope that it will whet your appetite to explore for yourself—in more depth—these amazing flowers.

> "O fleur-de-luce, bloom on, and let the river
> Linger to kiss thy feet;
> O flower of song, bloom on, and make forever
> The world more fair and sweet."
> —HENRY WADSWORTH LONGFELLOW

BACH FLOWER ESSENCES

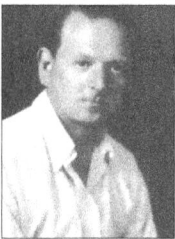

Dr. Edward Bach

In the early 1900s, Dr. Edward Bach trained at University College Hospital in England and held diplomas in public health, homeopathy, and bacteriology. During his work at the Royal London Homeopathic Hospital, Dr. Bach made an important discovery: those patients with the same emotional difficulties needed the same homeopathic treatment, irrespective of their physical illness. For Dr. Bach, these homeopathic treatments became the vehicle to rediscover the healing power of flower essences.

As a result of his newfound passion for energetic healing, Dr. Bach decided to leave his comfortable medical practice and move deep into the English countryside. It is here that he observed and intuited the flowers around him, discovering that each plant held an imprint that corresponded to a specific emotional state. Like the healers before him, Dr. Bach noted that the dew on the flowers became impregnated with the plant's healing properties. To re-establish what nature had shown him, he created a way to reproduce this dew, which resulted in the Bach Flower Essence family—seven groups of remedies that correspond to thirty-eight different negative states of mind. They represent "complimentary" remedies that can restore each one to a positive, natural state of harmony and well-being.

> *One month to the day before he died, Dr. Bach wrote:*
> "That there has been disclosed unto us a system of healing, such as has not been known within the memory of men; when, with the simplicity of the herbal remedies, we can set forth with the certainty, the absolute certainty, of their power to conquer disease."

Selected Bach Essences

Gentian

The Gentian flowers have opposite leaves and trumpet-shaped flowers that are usually deep blue or azure and generally grow in the Northern Hemisphere. There is little recorded history about this flower, but it is said that it was named after Gentius, King of Illyria, who used the flower for medical purposes. The origin of its meaning is not known, but it is sometimes referred to as the "disappointed gardener" since it can be temperamental to grow. Other names attributed to the humble gentian flowers are: you are unjust, loveliness, integrity, virgin pride, and intrinsic worth.

Since this Bach essence is used to help people who are easily discouraged and disheartened by setbacks, the definitions for Gentian take on both its positive and negative qualities. This delicate little flower helps to bring courage, optimism, and renewal through life's ups and downs.

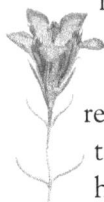

Emily Dickinson refers to the gentian flower in her poem number 442: "God made a little Gentian; It tried to be a Rose."

Olive

Even though the Olive leaf is mentioned in Genesis in the story of Noah and the great flood, it eventually became known as a symbol of peace. The historical record of Olive trees date back almost 6,000 years. The Olive tree is an evergreen with leaves that are bluish-green on top and white underneath. It thrives in lands with hot, dry summers and cool, damp winters. An Olive pit can grow into a tree that may live up to 1,000 years old. The Egyptians considered its branches to be a symbol of everlasting power, and the ancient Greeks used woven crowns of young Olive branches to celebrate winners of the first Olympic events. It is the distinctive dark, slim leaves of the Olive tree that are used in flower essences.

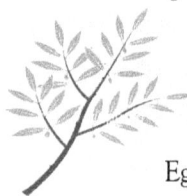

Olive Branch

Olive leaves have been shown to have significant antimicrobial action and are effective against many strong strains of fungi. As a flower essence, the energetic imprint of the long surviving Olive tree's leaf helps with renewal and regeneration and refreshes the spirit when one feels totally exhausted and has little strength to move on.

"They are beautiful. They are symbols of love. And their fragrance is a pleasure to the olfactory senses. However, along with all these qualities, flowers are also healers in their own right."
—DRS. RUPA AND ATUL SHAH

HIMALAYAN FLOWER ESSENCES

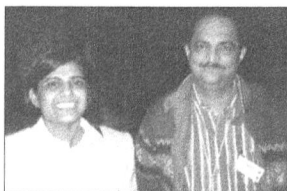

Drs. Rupa and Atul Shah

India has a very rich floral heritage. From the Himalayan foothills in the North to the tropical plains in the South, the extensive variety of flowering plants play a significant role in Ayurvedic medicine—a remarkable system that has been practiced continually for the past 5,000 years. This botanical backdrop is apparent throughout the Himalayan mountain range with its spectacular, uncorrupted landscape. Drs.

Rupa and Atul Shah, both allopathic doctors, became deeply interested in the history of Indian flower essences as an alternative therapy. They initially studied Bach Flower Essences, aromatherapy, and meditation, and then began to explore new flower essences harvested from the pristine slopes of the majestic Himalayas.

The Shah's opened two health centers where both orthodox and complementary methods are practiced, and they currently carry out in-depth research on the powerful balancing properties of recently developed flower essences. Using their scientific background and modern technology, they treat a wide variety of health issues—especially those related to stress—and they continue to research and record remarkable results.

Selected Himalayan Essences

Lotus

The Lotus Flower is a stout, creeping plant that grows in ponds and lakes. Its leaves grow above water level and are raised upward. The physical characteristics of this plant, with its beautiful blossom, reflect its spiritual symbolism and properties. The Lotus represents a classic "Doctrine of Signatures" example since it grows in the muddy, still water, yet its magnificent blossoms unfold, heaven bound, gradually, one petal at a time when touched by the rays of the morning sun. In Hindu lore, the mud in which the Lotus root grows represents material life, while the water through which the stalk passes represents the soul. When the plant reaches the surface of the water and opens its bud to the waiting sun, it represents the triumph of spirit over matter.

Throughout many spiritual traditions, the Lotus plant symbolizes spiritual illumination. In the Buddhist tradition, the fully opened Lotus has a strong, solar character and symbolizes enlightenment. Ancient Egyptian tradition held a similar interpretation and believed that meditating upon the Lotus flower brought harmony into all aspects of one's being, both internal and external.

The Lotus flower essence has many uses. It is known as a "spiritual elixir" since it helps to calm the mind, improve

"To keep the body in good health is a duty, for otherwise we shall not be able to trim the lamp of wisdom, and keep our mind strong and clear. Water surrounds the Lotus flower, but does not wet its petals."
—BUDDHA

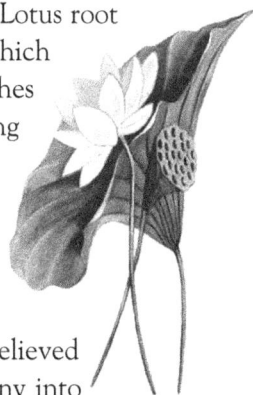

Lotus

concentration, and assist in spiritual growth. It also helps to correct emotional imbalances by allowing a gentle release of one's emotions. For example, a case of severe backache may be due to a suppressed stored emotion, and the Lotus essence can help to release this emotion through dreams. It is also a good harmonizing essence for interpersonal relationships, and can even enhance our ability to communicate with animals.

The Lotus flower essence can encourage recovery from illness, so it is ideally given to a patient at the start of therapy. It is also a very good aid to healers when diagnosing patients, especially when there is a doubt about which therapy to prescribe or when the patient's condition is confusing. Lotus essence has the unique ability to open one to a clearer understanding of the problem at hand. I often spray the room with *Lotus* and *Walnut* just before a flower essence therapy session to open up the channels of exploration.

Neem

This broad-leaved evergreen tree is thought to have originated in Northeast India; in the dry hills of Central India; and in Myanmar, Cambodia. Neem is often found growing in villages along the dusty roadside. The Neem tree could have been designed by a committee of genetic and chemical engineers, pharmacists, agronomists, and dieticians since its humble demeanor masks its many medicinal and therapeutic properties.

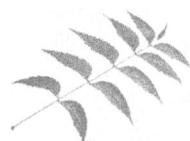

Neem Leaf

In 1922, British archaeologists discovered the now well-known 5,000-year-old Indus Valley site in Northwestern India. During their archaeological expeditions, they found skulls that had undergone cranial surgery, and clay pots that contained medicinal herbs. One of the most prominent of the medicinal herbs they found was *Azadirachta Indica*, also known as Neem.

The medicinal benefits of Neem are mentioned in the Veda's, a collection of one of the world's oldest spiritual texts. In India's ancient system of Ayurvedic medicine, every part of the Neem tree has been shown to promote health benefits. Traditionally, Neem has been an important remedy for blood purification and in the treatment of diabetes. One of the most well-known uses for Neem is in the prevention of tooth decay and gum disease. Neem twigs and leaves have been used for thousands of years by millions of people in India to brush their teeth, cleanse their gums, and to promote general oral hygiene. Even today, throughout India, in the morning light you can see people standing on the side of the road, brushing their teeth with a Neem twig.

The Neem flower essence helps to bring overly intellectual people into their hearts—making them more loving, more intuitive, less judgmental, more understanding, and more giving. This is why it is known as "the essence of the heart."

"The Bush Essences themselves have a tremendously important role to play. They are powerful catalysts for helping people heal themselves. These essences allow people to turn inward and understand their own life plan, their own life purpose and direction. They also give people the courage and confidence to follow that plan."
—IAN WHITE

AUSTRALIAN BUSH FLOWER ESSENCES

The Australian continent is a powerful and vibrant land whose energy has not been oversaturated by civilization, war, or pollution. The native Aborigines have acknowledged the power of flowers and have used them to heal emotional imbalances for many thousands of years. Many of the oldest flowers in world are found in the wilderness of the Australian Bush.

Ian White, a fifth-generation herbalist, spent much of his childhood bush-walking and learning about the healing properties

Ian White

of plants and flowers from his grandmother. Ian spent years imbibing and discovering the healing properties of many rare and unique flowers and is a celebrated flower essence practitioner. During meditation, he was shown pictures of certain plants and locations to harvest them. Along with his wife Kirsten, they developed over fifty Australian Bush Flower Essences that aid people in finding courage and strength in dealing with emotional challenges.

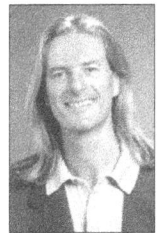

Sunshine Wattle

In the Australian Bush family, the Sunshine Wattle, also known as Acacias, is one of the most common and widespread of all Australian plants. It is derived from the thorny Egyptian tree known as *akakia*, and the common English name "wattle" means covering. This lovely plant inhabits the woodlands, dry forest, and rocky hillsides comprised of poor soil. Its bright, fluffy flowers are delightful to look at; the flower itself is actually a cluster of six to fifteen small flowers with long, pollen laden, yellow stamens.

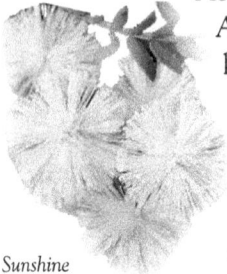

Sunshine Wattle

There are a number of interesting aspects of the Sunshine Wattle. It has evolved to adapt to the harsh, arid Australian climate and has the ability to survive long droughts. Its potent, protein-filled seeds were eaten by the early Aboriginal tribes, and the sturdy stems were used by the first scrubby fleet settlers in their buildings.

The Sunshine Wattle flower essence is often used as an aid during temporary difficulties, since it helps us move from the past into the present with determination. Its physical attributes strikingly resemble its nickname, "the optimistic essence."

Black-Eyed Susan

This is a favorite flower of many people. It grows wild almost everywhere, from roadsides to sprawling meadows. In the Australian countryside, the Black-Eyed Susan is unique. It is found on sandstone plateaus in the Sydney suburbs as well as in the dry forest and woodlands. The delicate blossoms grow on small, shrub-like plants and have petals that hang down like a bell. Susan's "black eyes" are filled with pollen.

This droopy flower has a prayerful pose and, when used as an essence, helps one to slow down and become more attuned to inner peace, gentleness, compassion, and intuition. However, in our contemporary and often hectic times, the Black-Eyed Susan's greatest asset is to relieve stress, which makes it a very valuable and timely essence, indeed.

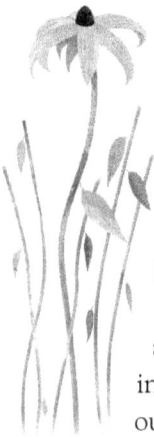

Black-Eyed Susan

"Flower essence therapy utilizes a precise understanding that the thoughts, feelings, and experiences of the human psyche are reflections of the same cosmic laws inherent in the growth patterns, shapes, colors, fragrances, and vital energies of nature which are expressed in the flowering plant."
—FLOWER ESSENCE SOCIETY

NORTH AMERICAN ESSENCES (FES)

The Flower Essence Society (FES), started by Patricia Kaminski and Richard Katz, has been in existence longer than any other flower essence organization other than Bach. Richard's early background was primarily in the field of science and mathematics. During that time, he also studied psychology, plant science, herbology, and flower essence therapy. Through years of study and practice, he became a pioneer in developing flower remedies from North American plants that were gathered from their pristine natural habitats in California and other parts of North America.

Richard Katz and Patricia Kaminski

Patricia, a gifted flower remedy practitioner, also studied widely and used flower remedies in the field of education. She joined Richard in starting the center to preserve and research this wisdom and also demonstrate the relationship between the human psyche and the healing properties in nature. Today, FES essences are used by thousands of practitioners in more than fifty countries around the world.

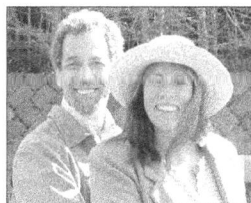

Selected FES Essences

Pretty Face
The Pretty Face flower is more commonly known as the Triplet Lily. It is native to the western parts of North America and, most commonly, in California. This perennial plant grows from a fibrous corm, which is a short, vertical, underground stem that serves as a storage organ, enabling the plant to survive adverse conditions such as summer drought and winter cold.

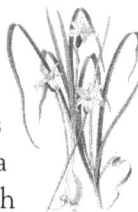

Triplet Lily

Triplet Lily get their name from the fact that all parts of their flowers come in threes. The "Pretty Face" name of this flower essence matches its properties, when in reality it is actually a very scrappy-looking plant and flower. However, the name makes perfect sense, since the essence is used for those with low self-esteem. Pretty Face is an ideal remedy for those whose spiritual light is caged, who live in anonymity—wallflowers, invisible in society. It is for people who have a hard time seeing their own beauty or who have not found their path of power and service. The Pretty Face flower essence helps shift the soul's awareness from looking outside itself by opening contact with its true inner luminosity—the real component of beauty.

Chamomile

Wild Chamomile is an annual herb that grows along fence rows, roadsides, and in sunny, open fields throughout southern Canada and into the northern U.S. The light green leaves are finely divided and covered with a down-like substance. In fact, when we lived in Nova Scotia, miniature daisy-like Chamomile clusters grew wild and abundant on the edges of our long, rocky driveway, fragranting the air with its soothing apple-pineapple scent.

Chamomile is one of the most loved and often-used herbs throughout history. Its name is derived from the Greek word "kamai melon," meaning "ground apple" due to its apple-like fragrance. The early Egyptians revered this herb for its effectiveness in curing chills caused by malaria. In fact, they dedicated Chamomile to their sun god, valuing its healing qualities over all other herbs. Because of its sedative and relaxing properties, Chamomile became an ingredient that was added to love potions during the middle ages. The Greek physician Dioscorides (first century AD), and Roman naturalist Pliny (23 AD), both advocated it for baths, warm poultices, relief of liver problems, bladder and kidney disorders, as well as for headaches. Chamomile was also used to refresh the air during a time when bathing was infrequent. Stems were strewn on the floor where they would release a pleasant fragrance when stepped on. In her charming 1902 classic, *Peter Rabbit*, Beatrix Potter wrote of a healing Chamomile tea that was given to the feverish Peter Rabbit by his mother.

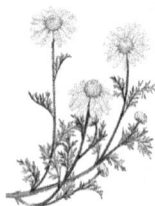

Chamomile

These very attributes make Chamomile an ideal flower essence when one is upset, moody, or irritable and helps to create a serene, sunny disposition by fostering emotional balance. This flower essence works on the "inner weather" when the emotional landscape is upset and filled with clouds. Chamomile can help one to see that the light is always peacefully shining regardless of outward events. It is particularly useful for people who have difficulty in letting go of emotional stress.

"These flower essences help us to open our eyes and see things as they really are; to let go of fears and to discover the real power that lies at the heart of each one of us; to discover more about ourselves than perhaps we ever dreamt possible . . . If, then, we are to find true happiness in this life, we need to discover our own true worth. It is here that the essences can help, suggesting to us how we need to change."
—ARTHUR BAILEY

BAILEY ESSENCES

Arthur Bailey, a scientist and chartered engineer, was always drawn to flowers. The catalyst that inspired him to enter the world of flower essences began after a serious bout with the flu and its significant cure by a homeopathic doctor. He began using Bach Flower Essences, and then, through meditative intuition, he discovered healing plants that grew from the fertile hills of Scotland to the Cornwall countryside. He found that these specific flower essences worked on the attitude of one's mind rather than on specific emotional issues. Bailey Essences are unique in their ability to integrate mind, body, and soul, while assisting in breaking through old conditioning and beliefs that limit our freedom.

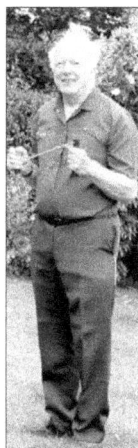

Arthur Bailey

Although Arthur Bailey passed away in 2008, Bailey Flower Essences continue to be a family dedication and passion. Based in the rural town of Ilkley within the Yorkshire Dales, most of the flowers that are used are still hand-picked from the Baileys' original garden.

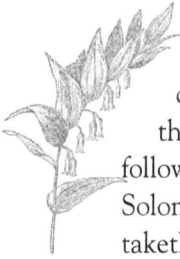

Solomon's Seal

Solomon's Seal has a long history of use in natural medicine dating back to the time of Dioscorides and Pliny. John Gerard, the noted herbalist and author of *Herball* (1597), wrote the following interesting passage about this flower: "The roots of Solomon's Seal, stamped while it is fresh and green and applied, taketh away in one night or two at the most, any bruise, black or blue spots."

Solomon's Seal

The bright green Solomon's Seal is a perennial native herb which is found growing in woods and thickets, in light shade or partial sun. The foliage is attractive, but the flowers are simple and not very showy. Their stems grow from a height of 18 inches to 2 feet and bend over gracefully. The light yellow-green flowers are tubular, succulent, thick and hang in delightful little drooping clusters of two to five.

My way of remembering the thick bunches of Solomon's Seal flowers is to associate them with a group of people sitting on benches, chatting away, their heads touching. It's an interesting visual since this flower essence is for those who are constantly busy. It can also be helpful for those who suffer from a babbling, restless mind and helps to restrain unruly thoughts.

Bistort

The name Bistort comes from the Latin *bis*, meaning "twice," and *torta*, meaning "twisted." This twisted, creeping plant is common in the north of England and grows in moist meadows in southern Scotland. The leaves and young shoots have been widely used in northern England as a well-known ingredient in herb pudding, and throughout the counties of Lancashire and Cumberland. Bistort is prepared as a green vegetable called *Patience Dock* and *Passions*, while the roots and leaves are used as a remedy for wounds. But the downfall of this plant is that when it becomes well-established, it often becomes a nuisance, especially in low-lying pastures; its root-stock forms large, well-extended patches and takes over the land.

Bistort

Like its root-stock, the Bistort flower essence is for those who find

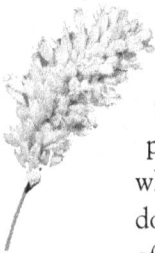

themselves overwhelmed and at a point in life that involves a major change. Bistort can help turn a breakdown into a breakthrough. It helps those who are unable to see the way forward and recognize a support system available from others and from within themselves. This remedy can be very empowering by helping people find the resolve and strength they need to rise above their current difficulties and make the necessary adjustments.

"The positive patterns of energy embodied in flower essences awaken dormant qualities of consciousness within us and stimulate the release of blockages to our spiritual evolution, which can be seen as the ongoing process of anchoring our spiritual selves into our physical bodies."
—STEVE JOHNSON

ALASKAN ESSENCES

Steve Johnson was a wilderness firefighter who worked in the remote interior of Alaska. It was there that he discovered the vibrational purity of the Alaskan countryside, where much of its pristine environment has remained untouched through the ages. The unspoiled forests and tundra regions, which are home to many distinctive species of plants, kindled Johnson's interest in the therapeutic use of flowers. He spent most of his time studying the names and uses of all the local plants and then began preparing them as flower essences. Johnson found that the native plants had adapted and flourished in a vibrant ecosystem of extremes that ranged from frigid cold to sweltering heat, and from long, dark winters to summers of perpetual light. These flowers reflect a special strength and vitality that are drawn from the land itself. Their unique properties are oriented toward healing the heart and relationships. They form an exceptional range of vibrational energy and healing qualities that are relevant to inner growth and the evolution of human consciousness.

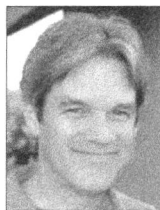

Steve Johnson

Foxglove

The lovely Foxglove thrives in areas with high concentrations of iron and coal. In fact, in the Soviet Union, prospectors looking for coal fields would simply search for fields of Foxglove. Their thimble-shaped flowers appear in the late spring sporting tall, pastel-colored spikes. Depending on the variety, their throats are generally white with mostly burgundy spots.

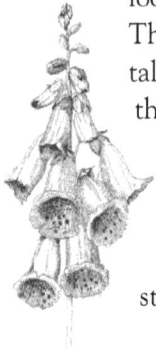

Although Foxglove can be very dangerous if misused, it has a long history of medicinal use for heart and kidney problems, edema, and aconite poisoning. Legend says that Vincent van Gogh used it to treat his epilepsy. An old saying about Foxglove states: "It can raise the dead and can kill the living."

Foxglove

In the 1700s, William Withering learned of this folk remedy from "an old woman in Shropshire," the West Midland region of England, and began studying its properties. This led to a search for the "active ingredient," which Withering found to be digitalis, the life-changing, plant-derived medicine that is currently used to treat a variety of heart problems.

The origin of the common name "Foxglove" is unclear, but it may refer to the folklore of faeries, since "folks glove" means the gloves of the folk (or fairies.) The Latin name, digitalis, comes from the word "digitanus," meaning "finger," because of the thimble shaped flowers that appears to cover a finger.

The unique power of this Alaskan flower essence lies in its ability to help release fear and emotional tension while enabling our perception to expand and connect with the truth of the situation we find ourselves in. It helps us to see our lack of perspective in dealing with a challenging situation, especially when we are unable to perceive the life lesson at the heart of a conflict or difficulty.

Valerian

Valerian is a hardy perennial flowering plant with heads of sweetly scented pink or white flowers. It has been used as a medicinal herb since the time of ancient Greece and Rome and during the tenth century by Arab physicians. Hippocrates described

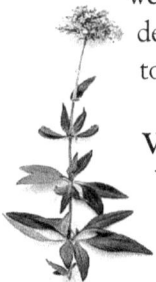

Valerian

its therapeutic uses in the second century, and Galen of Pergamum (Turkey) later prescribed it as a remedy for insomnia. In medieval Sweden, it was sometimes placed in the groom's wedding clothes to ward off the "envy" of the elves.

It is a derivative from the Latin word valere, meaning to "make strong," "being well," "feeling good," and "having a good morale." As a flower essence, the powerful Valerian plant helps us slow down so we may gain perspective on our priorities. It promotes peaceful relationships and helps different groups of people find common ground and harmony.

"Perfumes are the feelings of flowers."
—HEINRICH HEINE

AYURVEDIC ATTARS/ AROMATHERAPEUTIC EXTRACTS

The word attar is Persian/Arabic and means, "fragrance, scent, or essence." Attars have been used in the Near East, Persia, and India for over 5,000 years and are known as primary or foundation scents. Archaeological digs in ancient India have revealed round copper stills that were used for making attars; these stills are called *degs*. Following the seasons of the flowers, traditional attar-makers, with their

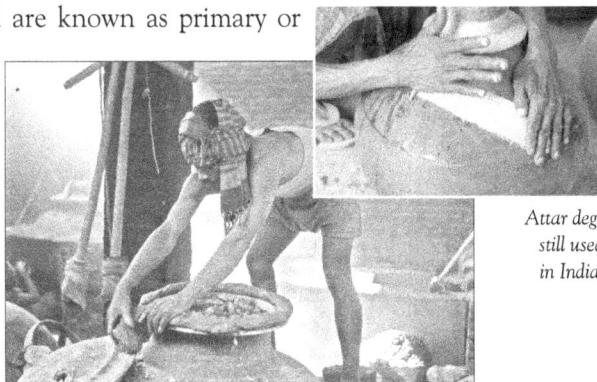

Attar degs still used in India.

degs, travelled all over India to make attars on the spot.

Utilizing similar techniques to the Indian attars, aromatherapeutic extracts use a variety of extracting techniques to capture the pure oil of plants. Beginning with ancient healers throughout the world, these fragrant oils were and continue to be used to enhance mood, adjust emotions, and uplift the soul. They are used to treat the whole person: physically, emotionally, and spiritually. They have a tremendous effect on the olfactory nerves: their healing properties form the foundation for the art of aromatherapy. Using aromatherapy and attars in conjunction with flower essences is a great marriage. They blend and work together in a perfect synergy.

Ayurvedic Attar

Sandalwood

The origin of Sandalwood is not known, but is probably native to the arc of islands in southeastern Indonesia. Some believe that it is native to southern India, but most agree that Sandalwood trees have been growing for more than 2,000 years. Sandalwood oil is distilled from the roots and heartwood of trees that take up to fifty to eighty years to reach full maturity. In a remarkably lengthy manufacturing process, used since ancient times, the mature Sandalwood trees are cut down then left to be eaten by ants, which consume all but the fragrant heartwood and roots. Every part of the heartwood is used, including the sawdust.

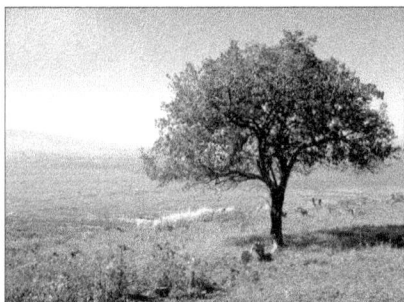

Indian Sandalwood Tree

The scent, called *chandana* in Sanskrit, is often used to induce a calm and meditative state. The fragrance actually improves with age. Throughout India and the Far East, temple gates and religious statues are carved from Sandalwood because of its spiritual association. The exquisite, long-lasting scent makes the wood impervious to termites and other insects. The southern Indian city of Mysore produces the finest quality oil, and the endangered Sandalwood trees are regulated by the Indian government.

When used as an Ayurvedic Attar, Sandalwood excels at heightening a sense of calm by fostering introspection and quieting the senses. Topically, Sandalwood oil is especially helpful on rashes, inflammation, acne, and dry or dehydrated skin.

Lavender

Lavender is native to the mountainous regions of the Mediterranean, where it grows in sunny, stony habitats. Today, it also grows throughout southern Europe, Australia, and the United States. The oil in Lavender's small, blue-violet flowers gives the herb its healing properties and fragrant scent.

Throughout history, Lavender has been known for its impressive healing powers. There are significant documented texts explaining its use throughout the past 2,500 years. In ancient times, Lavender was used for mummification as well as a perfume by the Egyptians, Phoenicians, and people of Arabia. The Romans used Lavender oil for bathing, cooking, and scenting the air, and they most likely coined its modern name from its Latin root, either lavare (to wash) or livendula (livid or bluish).

Lavender is mentioned often in the Bible, not by the modern name Lavender, but rather by its ancient name: *spikenard*. In the Gospel of Luke, it is recorded: "Then Mary took a pound of ointment of *spikenard*, very costly, and anointed the feet of Jesus and wiped his feet with her hair; and the house was filled with the odor of the ointment."

Throughout Medieval and Renaissance Europe, washer women were known as "lavenders" since they used Lavender to scent clothes and dry laundry on Lavender bushes. During that time, Lavender, along with other medicinal herbs, was often grown in "infirmarian's gardens," generally within monastery grounds. Hildegard von Bingen noted that Lavender "water"—a decoction of vodka, gin, or brandy mixed with Lavender—was helpful for treating migraine headaches.

Lavender is considered to be a natural remedy for a wide variety of ailments ranging from insomnia and anxiety to depression and

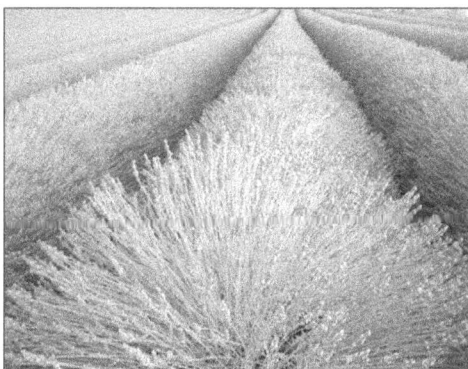

mood disturbances. Research has confirmed that Lavender is very effective in producing calming, soothing, and sedative effects.

Lavender makes a powerful aromatherapeutic extract. Among several fragrances tested by aromatherapy researchers, Lavender was found to be the most effective at relaxing brain waves and reducing stress. Interestingly, it also reduced computer errors by almost one-fourth when used to scent the office. Lavender works on emotional issues to help break dogmatic patterns while encouraging one to deepen into spirit.

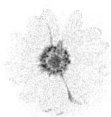

Chapter Seven
CASE STUDIES

"The noblest pleasure is the joy of understanding."
—LEONARDO DA VINCI

DIAGNOSTIC TOOLS

Throughout the decades, my experience as a practitioner has revealed the many diverse gifts and qualities that flower essences have to offer. In this chapter, I share a few stories in the hope that you may gain some insight into the dynamic process of diagnosing and using flower essences for yourself.

Regardless of the challenge, I find that, in most cases, flower essences always affect change in a variety of ways such as attitude, emotion, mood, or mental perception. As an integral therapy, it begins the healing process from the inside out.

You may recognize some of the challenges documented here in yourself or in someone you know. The healing combinations are as varied as the challenges themselves; they ideally complement the personality behind the problem. When working with flower essences, you can refer to some hands-on tools: exercises in Chapter Four to begin the discovery and treatment process, the Flower Essence Selection Guide on page 106; and a diagnostic form on page 137.

"Every human being is the author of his own health or dis-ease."
–BUDDHA

"Treat people as if they were what they ought to be, and you help them to become what they are capable of being."
—GOETHE

"A retired husband is often a wife's full-time job."
—ELLA HARRIS

The Case of the Nervous Retiree

Leon is an older gentleman who spent his life as a high-pressure executive in the fashion industry. After retiring from a hectic New York City lifestyle, he ended up moving to Florida where, rather suddenly, his pace of life slowed down to a crawl. Leon's only problem is that his mind didn't slow down to accommodate his new lifestyle. Even though, for the first time in his life, he had time on his hands, he continued to rush from one activity to the next. Leon hardly had the patience to sit at a red light. Mealtime was the worst: he would push everyone to hurry up for dinner, yet, as soon as they sat down for a relaxing meal, he would quickly eat in order to begin planning the next activity. He was a warm and friendly person, but also an incessant talker who would get right up in your face. Leon simply didn't have the ability to enjoy the relaxed lifestyle that a comfortable retirement afforded him.

Leon's wife tried everything to help him slow down and enjoy his new life. When she spoke with him about using flower essence therapy, he vehemently objected. So, I enlisted his wife to try a clandestine approach by slipping the prescribed flower essences into his orange juice each morning. The combination addressed his extreme impatience, the overall dramatic changes in his life, and his overactive personality.

About a week into Leon's "spiked" orange juice, his wife began to notice small changes. For example, the next time they decided to go out for dinner, he didn't stand by the door, pacing while she was getting ready. And, while sitting in traffic, he was able to laugh and comment about it rather than simply react. As time went on, the reports were more and more promising. Leon was finally allowing himself to adjust to his new, slower pace while feeling much more relaxed. He never knew that his morning glass of orange juice contained a life-changing remedy.

PROFILE
Primary Issues: Can't relax, talks too much, doesn't adjust to change.
Emotion/State of Mind: Restless, anxious, seeks attention, resistance.
Manifests As: Impatience, hyperactivity, inflexibility.
Positive Aspects: Hard worker, friendly, funny, curious, intelligent.

Treatment: Drops
Bach
> *Impatiens:* Helps a "type A" person become more patient and tranquil.
> *Walnut.* Helps one adjust to major life changes.
> *Heather:* Helps one to be a better listener and not so self-absorbed.

Bailey
> *Bistort:* Helps one to not be so vulnerable during major life changes and transitions. Fosters encouragement and acceptance.
> *Solomon's Seal:* This helps one to relax, to stop and smell the roses; quiets the restless mind.

Australian Bush
> *Black-Eyed Susan:* Especially helpful for the constant need to rush around; it helps one find inner calm.
> *Bottlebrush:* Helps to work through resistance to change, holding onto the past, and old habits which often affect seniors.

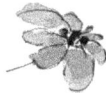

"Three Rules of Work: Out of clutter find simplicity; From discord find harmony; In the middle of difficulty lies opportunity."
—ALBERT EINSTEIN

The Case of Inner and Outer Clutter
Obsessive personalities often exhibit physical symptoms that match their mental states, and Penny's case was no exception. She suffered

from chronic neck pain that radiated down her arm. At first, she just wanted the pain to go away and visited a host of doctors, all of whom would invariably tell her, "It's all in your head." Penny became more and more discouraged and despondent.

When I first met Penny, I was impressed by her kindness, gentleness, and motherly demeanor, but as we investigated her situation together (something her doctors never thought to do), and went through her life history, it became apparent that she was a hoarder. She had a difficult time letting go of things, both physically and emotionally. Penny stored everything: from ideas and concepts, to clothing and magazines, to old pots and pans. Penny could never understand, nor even acknowledge, her habit of holding on to the past and her extreme attachment to possessions. She felt everything in her outer life was in control as long as she kept her stuff neatly sorted in closets, carefully piled up in the garage, or saved in cartons in a spare room. When we examined it closely, both her mind and her house were indeed cluttered. This hidden "clutter" reflected her personality and eventually spilled out into physical problems. Penny hid her challenges behind a smiling face so that even her closest friends didn't know the extent of her inner pain. Shining a light on the problem finally brought it out into the open.

I gave Penny a combination of essences for this particular personality trait that included hiding her feelings, obsessive behavior, and ongoing control issues. In a few weeks, Penny was able to begin the process of throwing away some of the stuff she never needed in the first place, and her mind, as a result, became clearer. She soon was able to admit to close friends that everything in her life was not what it appeared to be.

Penny had never learned how to untangle her attachment to relatively meaningless thoughts and objects. By working through this issue, layer by layer, she began to address the core problem. This was Penny's big challenge: to learn how to accept change and move beyond it. This was indeed a stubborn challenge since she revealed to me that her mother faced this issue as well. In fact, Penny's mother unintentionally taught her this dysfunctional behavior. Life changes simply paralyzed her; they rocked her safe world. For this deep-seated issue, I gave her a combination cream for accepting life changes. The breakthrough came a while after Penny began the new therapy, which she took each morning and evening. When Penny was finally able to acknowledge the patterns of her debilitating conditioning, little by little, her neck pain disappeared along with other symptoms. She began to consciously awake each morning to a new day and learned to appreciate life without holding on to it— either by defining it through the past or anticipating its unknown future.

PROFILE

Primary Issues: Inability to let go, hides feelings, difficulty accepting change, hoarder, cluttered mind.

Emotion/State of Mind: Shame, fear, resistance, obsession.

Manifests As: Possessiveness, frustration, being overwhelmed, discouragement.

Positive Aspects: Kind, gentle, makes others happy.

TREATMENT: Drops

Bach

Gentian: For the daily ups and downs, the little discouragements. When one is pre-wired to take even little things to heart and unable to let go of them. Uplifts one's spirits.

Agrimony: This essence works for those who mask their true feelings behind a smiling face, dulling themselves through obsessions.

White Chestnut: This helps one overcome overly scattered and persistent thought patterns, when one is unable to concentrate on the matter at hand.

Chicory: Ideal for the classic case of over-possessiveness, a clingy and "mothering" type of personality.

Australian Bush

Boronia: An excellent essence to help with obsessive behavior, regaining perspective, and fostering balance.

Bach

Walnut: This essence is used to help one open up to major life changes. It is given to help break free from old, stuck positions, and to establish new, healthier patterns.

Bailey

Bistort: A good partner with *Walnut* for major life changes and transitions, especially those in need of a breakthrough.

Australian Bush

Sunshine Wattle: Helps one perceive life as brighter and lighter, less unencumbered and trapped in the past; roots one in the present.

Bottlebrush: This essence is given to those overwhelmed by an enormous workload and in the process of turning one's life around, but not knowing how or where to begin.

Boab: For those who adopt family thought-patterns, repeating negative experiences from the past.

Aromatherapeutic Extract

Musk: This essential oil is good for vitality and focus.

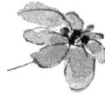

"The key to change is to let go of fear."
—ROSANNE CASH

The Case of the Attached Daughter

Jennifer is an extremely intelligent, creative, funny, and sensitive child, but she was overly attached to her parents. As an only child, she often fretted about their safety and well-being, which only increased when she went off to college. This was an interesting role reversal since it's parents who generally worry about their children when they leave the nest. During her first semester, this attachment began to impact both her health and studies. She began to have headaches and stomach upsets. Even though Jennifer was very bright, she had a hard time concentrating during her classes and became overly worried about her health. Jennifer's mother, a close friend of mine, asked for my advice. We talked for a while and I found out that, although Jennifer was a fairly sheltered child, she had never exhibited these symptoms to this extent before. In high school she was outgoing, confident, and popular.

This major change triggered a deeply held anxiety; Jennifer kept glamorizing her life in high school and wasn't able to appreciate her new life in college. She agreed to try a special cream mixture that she would use twice daily. She said that she liked the way it smelled and soon discovered, little by little, that she felt more comfortable being away from home. After some time, Jennifer revealed that she still had trouble focusing; the college environment was simply more distracting than what she was used to. I made up a new cream mixture by removing some of the original essences and adding new ones to address "focus" and "confidence." This did the trick. Slowly, Jennifer's physical problems began to dissipate. Although she struggled during her freshman year, she sailed through the following three years of school and eventually graduated with honors. Her mother truly believes that these flower creams made Jennifer's college experience a positive and wonderful time for her.

PROFILE
Primary Issues: Overly attached to family, easily distracted, concerned with health issues.
Emotion/State of Mind: Worry, frustration, fear, anxiety.
Manifests As: Oversensitivity, exhaustion, head and stomachache.
Positive Aspects: Smart, creative, witty.

TREATMENT: Cream
Bach
> *Red Chestnut:* This essence helps one to "let go" and move on. It addresses one's overconcern for family matters; it may manifest as physical problems and feelings of anxiety.
> *White Chestnut:* Used to calm an overactive mind filled with worry, "the escalator essence."

Crab Apple: The cleansing remedy. Helpful for ongoing obsession with health and poor self-image.

Honeysuckle: Helps support one's preoccupations with the past, a deep homesickness; to help one move into the present.

Australian Bush

Little Flannel Flower: An ideal remedy to help regain a natural sense of playfulness, humor, and spontaneity.

Wild Potato Bush: This essence gives one a sense of freedom and the ability to move on, unburdened and less restrictive.

Californian (FES)

Chamomile: When one is under stress, which can create stomach and headaches, this helps to regain one's carefree and happy nature.

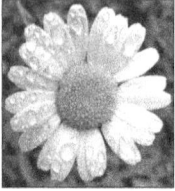

Chamomile

Aromatherapeutic Extract:

Frankincense: Helps to calm the body and overcome fear

Jasmine: Promotes peace, encourages openness and acceptance.

Added to Second Batch

Bach

Scleranthus: Especially helps to develop decisiveness, flexibility and concentration and relieves mood swings; brings thoughts into focus.

Larch: Builds one's sense of confidence and self-reliance; helps one to be bolder by plunging into life.

Australian Bush

Five Corners: This essence helps one celebrate inner beauty and acceptance of themselves, thereby increasing vitality.

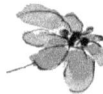

"Choose a job you love and you'll never work a day in your life."
—CONFUCIUS

The Case of Overresponsibility

Linny is an overly responsible person; at this particular time in her life, she became very unhappy at work. It simply didn't challenge her anymore, nor was she able to use her innate creative abilities. The job simply left her exhausted at the end of the day. Being a single mom, Linny couldn't take the financial risk of changing professions, yet she was always tired and irritable, frequently becoming ill; her immune system significantly compromised. Flower essences couldn't help Linny find a new job, but they could help reveal her options with a clearer perspective. Linny knew that if she didn't change her job, the stress might spiral into even worse health issues, and that her irritability was causing friction with her teenage son, limiting her ability to help him through his own problems.

I made a flower essence formula in a dropper bottle and asked Linny to sip it slowly throughout the day. She always had a bottle of water with her so she added several drops to the bottle and began to take it regularly. When her fear of change began to lessen and her mind became clearer, she earnestly began to research different types of work. Linny eventually identified three specific career areas she wanted to explore. The next step was to find the courage and confidence to put her research into practice, so we added two more essences to help her address this issue. Linny was soon preparing to interview for a job with a much greater sense of confidence and ease. She eventually found a job that allowed her to express her talent in crafts and also support her love of nature; she became an art counselor for the regional YMCA camp. The first week of her new job, almost miraculously, her enthusiasm and energy returned.

PROFILE
Primary Issues: Overwhelmed by responsibility, lack of confidence.
Emotion/State of Mind: Irritable, confused, fearful.
Manifests As: Exhaustion, emotionally drained, short-tempered.
Positive Aspects: Responsible, creative, enthusiastic.

TREATMENT: Drops
Issue One
Bach
Elm: For temporarily feeling overwhelmed and worn out. *Elm* helps one return to one's natural self-reliance and vibrant confidence.

Gentian: For discouragements, frustrations, doubts, and setbacks during one's day-to-day challenges.

Wild Oat: This helps when one is uncertain during the crossroads of life. Helps one uncover innate talents and vocational abilities.

Californian (FES)
Nasturtium: Helpful for a depleted life force and lack of emotional verve. Helps get one back to their radiant energy and a natural enthusiasm for whatever life brings.

Chamomile: The stress releaser.

Alaskan
Opium Poppy: Clears deep exhaustion, helps to integrate one's experiences and life lessons and live more fully in the present, restoring a sense of balance.

Issue Two
Bach
Larch: This essence is used to help with confidence and fear of failure, helps not to let life's opportunities pass one by.

Australian Bush
Bush Fuchsia: Along with *Larch*, this essence helps to boost self-confidence, clarity in public speaking, and is especially good during interviews.

> *"Each man has his own vocation; his talent is his call.*
> *There is one direction in which all space is open to him."*
> —RALPH WALDO EMERSON

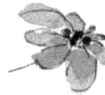

"Sometimes it's the smallest decisions that can change your life forever."
—KERI RUSSELL

The Case of the Overprotective Mother

Noreen was a good mother—actually a great mother—but perhaps *too much* of a mother. Her mind was either on her grown children and their problems or her grandchildren and their problems. This sense of overconcern impacted her ability to fully live her own life. She often spoke of what she wanted for her life, but lately, even this desire was subjugated by endless family worries. Finally, in a state of mental exhaustion, Noreen said she really just wanted peace of mind. And that was an excellent place to start. From a young age she was drawn to spirituality, and this aspect of her life was being ignored by waves of endless involvement.

Noreen started with a selection of four flower essences that addressed her need to "fix" everything for those she loved, her inability to say "no," and her increasing mental and physical exhaustion.

Little by little, Noreen began to step away from the heavy burden she had taken upon herself: the role of overseer in everyone else's life but her own! The second issue that flower essences addressed was the reconnection with Noreen's spiritual inclination.

After adding an additional four essences, she was able to re-direct her interest in spirituality by creating a group that gathered in her home to reflect on spiritual themes. Noreen was eventually able to live the life she had always envisioned for herself: fulfilling her own needs while interacting with family members with compassion, yet without excessive involvement.

PROFILE

Primary Issues: Overconcern for others, mental exhaustion, difficulty saying no.

Emotion/State of Mind: Worry, conflict, fear.

Manifests As: Possessiveness, disconnectedness, emotionally depleted.

Positive Aspects: Spiritual, maternal, kind, selfless.

TREATMENT: Drops

Issue #One

Bach

Red Chestnut: The perfect candidate for this essence is one who worries and obsesses about their loved ones; it helps to puts one's mind at rest.

Centaury: This essence is ideal for the kind-hearted person who puts themselves last and are unable to say "no" to anything. They often overextend and exhaust themselves by accommodating others, "people pleasers."

Olive: Endless worry can create great exhaustion and weariness; *Olive* is helpful to restore extreme depleted energy.

Australian Bush

Old Man Banksia: As an aboriginal symbol of female spirituality, this essence helps with low energy when one needs a pick-me-up and helps to renew a sense of enthusiasm.

Issue #Two

Bach

Larch: Helps one redirect one's life; gives one the confidence to fulfill one's dreams and not stand in the shadows.

Bailey

Almond: This essence is "the supportive inner teacher," which helps us to reconnect with our soul and encourages intuition.

Australian Bush Remedies

Red Grevillea: This essence helps people who are overly sensitive and feeling stuck, when one knows their goal but not how to get there. Helps one break free and establish independence; encourages boldness.

Himalayan

Lotus: This is a unique flower essence that assists in spiritual growth; balances and cleanses while aiding one in meditation.

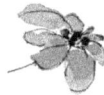

"Behold, I show you a mystery; we shall not all sleep, but we shall all be changed, in a moment, in the twinkling of an eye."
—CORINTHIANS

The Case of Endless Menopause

Michelle came to me during a ten-year battle with menopause. She had tried everything: hormone replacement therapy, bioidentical hormones, acupuncture, herbal supplements—you name it. Strong allopathic medicines didn't suit her and herbal supplements didn't work! Everything she understood about menopause led her to understand that her symptoms were lasting a very long time. So, when we sat down, Michelle exclaimed, "I'm just exhausted by this!" She meant both, physically and emotionally. She also felt overly sensitive about everything in her life, along with the extra weight gain that came with menopause and the effect it had on her appearance and confidence.

Michelle's temperament was artistic and easy-going, so we used essences that would complement her personality. Michelle was eager to try anything. I made a healing cream for her to use before sleep and asked her to check back with me in a few weeks. Michelle phoned three weeks later, quite cheerful and chatty, and she said that she finally felt "up" and was beginning to feel full of life again. With the help of the cream, Michelle was able to go back to sleep after being awakened by a hot flash, and she no longer fretted over these occurrences.

PROFILE
Primary Issues: Exhausted, tired, worn-out.
Emotion/State of Mind: Frustrated, annoyed, bitter.
Manifests As: Distress, impatience, melancholy.
Positive Aspects: Creative, calm, optimistic.

TREATMENT: Drops

Bach

Crab Apple: Cleanses the body and mind. Helps with issues of personal self-image.

Californian (FES)

Chamomile: Helps regain inner peace, harmony, and a sense of humor.

Australian Bush

She Oak: This essence is used to treat female hormone imbalances and is often the first remedy to draw on for any hormonal issue. Helps with fluid retention.

Macrocarpa: Helps revive one's body after years of experiencing exhaustion; to regenerate the adrenal glands as well as renew enthusiasm and inner strength.

Bottlebrush: Especially helpful during the various stages of menopause.

Old Man Banksia: Helps with weight issues, when one feels bogged down, sluggish.

TREATMENT: Cream

(Along with the remedies above, two more remedies and two aromatherapeutic extracts were combined in a cream base.)

Bailey

White Dead Nettle: Similar to *White Chestnut,* this helps stop one's revolving thoughts and fixation about one's long-term condition. Gives one a break from the endless cycle of thought patterns.

Californian (FES)

Saint John's Wort: Helpful for sensitive, fair-skinned people prone to environmental stress. This essence helps to give protection, strength and illumined consciousness, especially at night.

Aromatherapeutic Extract

Amber: This aromatherapy extract helps to stabilize the endocrine system and promotes balance.

Lavender: With its lovely scent, *Lavender* is especially helpful for sleep issues.

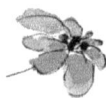

"If you ask what is the single most important key to longevity,
I would have to say it is avoiding worry, stress, and tension.
And if you didn't ask me, I'd still have to say it."
—GEORGE F. BURNS

The Case of Runaway Stress

Most people know that stress is dangerous, even deadly. However, knowing this doesn't necessarily mean one assimilates its implication. Although Nick is a natural optimist, a good husband, provider, and attentive father, at this junction in his life, there were several challenges that caused his productivity to slow down enormously. This, in turn, created financial havoc, which spiraled into restlessness and insomnia—a domino effect that created even more stress and isolation, all of which he couldn't share with friends. The combination of emotional triggers created a vicious circle: lack of sleep heightened his problems and caused even more sleeplessness—it just went on and on. Nick was on the cusp of an acute mid-life crisis.

Luckily, Nick had the support of his wife. At first, she wasn't sure if Nick would consider using flower essences, but when she approached him, he embraced the concept, longing for any relief he could get. During his first excursion into the world of flower essences, we worked on a foreboding sense of "doom and gloom" that would overtake him. After the first two weeks, he began to feel more open to life's possibilities. Later, as his mind began to clear, Nick started to see a way out of the emotional maze that he found himself in.

Change was always an issue for Nick, yet change was exactly what he needed. However, the change was not necessary in his profession, but rather, a change of attitude. This approach took some time to absorb. When Nick was able to sleep better, clarity began to return and he was able to use this experience as a stepping-stone to transform his outlook. The next step was to remove some of the initial essences and introduce new ones. This change helped Nick see light, in what was previously darkness. It was quite an evolution.

Nick began living one day at a time and experienced the glass of his life as half-full rather than half-empty. This change in attitude helped Nick control the stress that was a threat to his body and mind. He was able to move forward with renewed energy and could appreciate all that he had worked so hard to achieve. While this is an ongoing challenge for him, the flower essences are available when he needs to be refreshed or recharged. It reminds him to maintain perspective and hold on to the true blessings that surround him.

PROFILE
Primary Issues: Sleeplessness, financial insecurity, despair, stress.
Emotion/State of Mind: Overwhelmed, fearful, anxious.
Manifests As: Restlessness, negativity, despondent.
Positive Aspects: Responsible, optimistic, attentive.

TREATMENT: Drops
Issue One
> **Bach**
>> *Mustard:* For deep gloom which descends without any specific reason.
>> *White Chestnut:* Helps in quieting and calming the mind before sleep.
> **Bailey**
>> *Solomon's Seal:* Since this essence helps to clear the mind, it allows one to not get bogged down by trivia and begin to see life's true purpose.
> **Himalayan**
>> *Ashoka Flower:* Helps with deep-seated disharmony and isolation.
> **Australian Bush**
>> *Bottlebrush:* Like *Walnut*, it is helpful during crucial life changes.
> **Alaskan**
>> *Lamb's Quarter:* Heals isolation; brings mind and heart into balance.
> **Californian (FES)**
>> *Chamomile:* The "stress buster" essence when emotional balancing is needed; restores one's sunny disposition.

Bach

Gentian: This essence helps when one lacks faith in their ability to succeed; keep one's spirits upbeat through the day.

Australian Bush

Sunshine Wattle: Helps with temporary hopelessness and worry, especially about one's financial position; helps one see a bright future.

Little Flannel Flower: The "child within us" essence; helps one lighten up, become more playful and spontaneous.

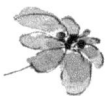

"The appearance of a disease is swift as an arrow;
its disappearance slow, like a thread."
—CHINESE PROVERB

The Heart of the Case

Donald is an elderly man who recently underwent an angiogram of the heart. To close the incision (which was made to access one of the main arteries leading to the heart) on the upper part of his thigh, a device called an *angioplug* was used. The angioplug was developed to save time in closing the incision and also to avoid an overnight hospital stay.

However, for Donald, the angioplug didn't work that well and caused some blood leakage, which created a huge black and blue wound down his thigh, almost to his knee. The wound was painful and made it difficult for Don to walk, and he was continually tired throughout the day. Though Donald was a quiet, patient, and peaceful person who didn't often complain, he was growing frustrated that this seemingly routine procedure was taking so long to heal.

I decided to try a combination of remedies that work well in healing skin injuries. Although cream is applied topically, this remedy also works on emotional issues. Don began to apply this cream every morning and every evening. Each morning, when he awoke, he noticed an improvement in the wound.

On the few days that he forgot to use the cream, the wound

"The heart has reasons that reason cannot know."
–BLAISE PASCAL

remained the same, with almost no improvement. Within two weeks, the large black and blue patch, physical discomfort, and emotional disturbance began to diminish, and his normal happy demeanor returned.

PROFILE
Primary Issues: Bruising, trauma to the skin.
Emotion/State of Mind: Impatient, resentful.
Manifests As: Frustration, uncomfortable feeling.
Positive Aspects: Peaceful, cheerful, romantic.

TREATMENT: Cream
Bach
Gentian: This essence is given for daily discouragement.
Crab Apple: Cleanses the body and mind; works on the overconcern of physical issues and negative perceptions of our body.
Star of Bethlehem: Helps when there is any shock or trauma to the body.
Alaskan
Foxglove: This helps stimulate the release of fear and emotional tension around the heart. During difficulties, enables one to accept the reality of the situation one finds oneself in.
Himalayan
Neem: This is an essence of the heart, which is appropriate for anyone with heart issues.
Ashoka Flower: For those who have gone through great trauma due to a specific event. It has a positive effect on elderly people; helps to create an atmosphere of harmony and well-being.
Australian Bush
Spinifex: This empowers one, through emotional understanding, to heal physical conditions. Works well topically, especially on bruises, surface cuts, and lesions.

Aromatherapeutic Extract
Ylang Ylang: This is known for its unique relationship to the heart; it can be used to help alleviate the symptoms of shock and trauma.
Rose: Rose is used as a tonic for the heart and for emotional upliftment.

"You, yourself, as much as anybody in the entire universe,
deserve your love and affection."
—BUDDHA

The Case of Childhood Trauma

Franny was adopted at an early age, she is now ten, but due to early trauma she experiences a wide range of emotional issues, beginning with feelings of deep frustration, attention-seeking, and impulsivity.

In public places she has a hard time controlling her behavior, which often ends up in a two-year-old type of tantrum, resulting in Fanny's mom physically removing her from the scene and taking her home. Another issue is that she has a hard time getting to sleep and waking up in the morning.

Since Franny is under the care of a family physician, I asked her mother if she would like to try a flower essence cream combination as a complimentary therapy. Franny's mother was happy to try this natural treatment, especially since she understood it wouldn't interfere with Franny's comprehensive medication regime. So, she began to apply the cream daily, especially just before bed. She found that Franny was able to fall asleep quicker and wake up easier. But since her emotional issues are quite deep-seated this continues to be a work in progress.

I added essences to treat her long-term issues and Franny's mother has noticed that, when a situation arises and the cream is used, Franny is able to handle the situation better and it often comes to resolution quicker.

PROFILE
Primary Issues: Craves attention, impulsive.
Emotion/State of Mind: Anger, obsessiveness.
Manifests As: Animosity, aggression, occasional feelings of acute distress.
Positive Aspects: Curious, athletic, artistic, and funny.

TREATMENT: Cream
Bach
White Chestnut: Helps the restless mind by giving one a break from endless thoughts, allowing the mind to function clearly and efficiently.

Cherry Plum: This is used to address more extensive and extreme emotional issues when one is unable to control one's thoughts and may be impulsive.

Chestnut Bud: This essence is good for one who has a challenging time learning from past lessons; helps stop endless patterns of repeating mistakes.

Holly: Holly is used to help mitigate feelings of bitterness, envy, and jealousy.

Californian (FES)
Morning Glory: For night owls who have erratic sleep rhythms and difficulty getting up in the morning; helpful for imbalance, especially when one is not able to fully be at home in one's body and has a depleted life force.

Australian Bush
Boronia: This essence is often prescribed to resolve obsession with thoughts, events, and things and when one has detachment issues. It helps one move toward clarity and focus.

Himalayan
Peacock Flower: This essence is for anyone who needs to be rehabilitated from long, debilitating physical and mental problems; opens the channel to restore energy flow.

Aromatherapeutic Extract:
Honeysuckle: This extract helps with fear and sadness, creating a circle of safety and love.

"Anxiety is the space between the "now" and the "then."
—RICHARD ABELL

The Case of Unknown Fear

Holly is a highly sensitive person with a serious interest in spirituality. She suddenly began waking up from a deep sleep and experiencing a sense of foreboding and panic. There was no known reason for this, it was just a vague and shadow-like fear. Her heart would race and she couldn't get back to sleep. It was obvious that Holly needed to restore healthy sleep patterns and address the anxiety and panic that resulted from these events. Specific flower essences were combined into a cream base to help her overcome this unknown fear. Holly used the cream until this period finally passed. She also knew that if help was needed again, the cream was available in her medicine cabinet. This gave her an additional sense of comfort and relief.

PROFILE

Primary Issues: Sleeplessness, overly sensitive, fear.
Emotion/State of Mind: Anxiety, panic, terror.
Manifests As: Disconnectedness, restless thoughts.
Positive Aspects: Spiritual, kind, open to healing.

TREATMENT: Cream

Bach

White Chestnut: Helps one sleep soundly and not dwell on thoughts of panic and apprehension.

Aspen: Helpful when the fear is of unknown, irrational, and vague origin; when it descends like a blanket or dense fog.

Rock Rose: Helps with trembling feeling, fear, panic, and terror.

Californian (FES)

Saint John's Wort: This essence is helpful for night terrors and to illuminate one's consciousness, especially for oversensitive souls.

Himalayan

Lotus: Helps one reconnect with one's spiritual self; clears toxins.

Ayurvedic Attar

Sandalwood: This attar has a lovely scent that helps promote peace.

"An old cat will not learn how to dance."
—Moroccan Proverb

The Case of the Loud Cat

At the same time Linny (page 69) was undergoing the challenge of discovering her vocation, her cat, Screecher, was going through his own emotional problems. They had recently moved into a new apartment, which they now shared with another cat. Coming into another cat's territory can be quite a challenge, and this was especially difficult for Screecher. Even though he is generally a calm, if not reserved cat, he is also well-named since his voice is shrill and loud. Because he was used to being king of his own castle, Screecher started acting out, doing what he did best: screech—especially at night when Linny needed her rest. I made up a combination bottle of essences and told Linny to put it in Screecher's food bowl. At first, the fussy and intuitive cat knew something was up and stopped eating. So we went to Plan B. We put the essences in a spray bottle, and Linny sprayed him several times each day. After two nights, Screecher and Linny began to relax and started to get some sleep.

PROFILE

Primary Issues: Demanding, spoiled, craves attention, talkative.
Emotion/State of Mind: Anger, jealousy, frustration.
Manifests As: Animosity, displeasure, restlessness.
Positive Aspects: Calm, reserved, attentive.

TREATMENT: Spray

Bach

Walnut: Helps reduce resistance to a life issue or change.
Heather: This is the classic remedy for those who are overly talkative.
Holly: Helps with feelings of envy and jealousy.
Beech: Helps with irritability and intolerance of others.

Bailey

Solomon's Seal: Helps relaxation, slowing down and becoming quieter.

Californian (FES)

Chamomile: Releases emotional tension, which can lead to moodiness and restlessness; helps to become more serene and emotionally balanced.

"Ring the bells that still can ring.
Forget your perfect offering.
There is a crack in everything.
That's how the light gets in."
—LEONARD COHEN

The Case of the Perfectionist

Jim is an efficient and creative person; he dots all his "i's" and crosses all his "t's," and any employer would love to hire him. The only problem is that he became exhausted, experienced panic attacks, and suffered from headaches. If anything in life was not as perfect as Jim demanded, he simply couldn't handle it. He generally procrastinated when beginning a new project until everything was in perfect order. One of his friends recommended that he see me since recent medical tests didn't show anything physically wrong with him. While speaking with Jim, it was obvious that he controlled his world. When unexpected twists of life occurred, as they often do, he would collapse into a state of self-created misery, which affected him both physically and mentally. He said he liked being a perfectionist, though he didn't think of himself as controlling.

Since he was open to trying flower essences, we began with a specific combination. Amazingly, within days, Jim began to relax and allow himself a tiny break from his rigidity. It took a month before he was able to acknowledge and give voice to some of his own imperfections. He soon began accepting the uncontrollable events in his life without overreacting, and stopped obsessing about unrealistic hopes and dreams. We continue to work together on new issues as they appear.

PROFILE
Primary Issues: Headaches, panic attacks, intensity.
Emotion/State of Mind: Anxiety, exhaustion, obsession, procrastination.
Manifests As: Resistance, rigidity, unhappiness.
Positive Aspects: Responsible, creative, intelligent.

Treatment: Drops

Bach

Rock Rose: Helps with trembling feeling, fear, panic, and terror.

Vine: For inflexibility; unrealistic expectations of oneself and others.

Hornbeam: Procrastination, exhaustion at the thought of beginning a new project.

Alaskan

Wild Rhubarb: For mental inflexibility; encourages and balances the rational and intuitive.

Australian Bush

Bauhinia: For embracing new concepts; for people set in their ways.

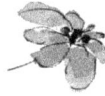

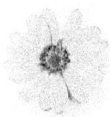

Chapter Eight

FLOWER ESSENCE STUDIES

*"The most beautiful plants and herbs to be found in the
pharmacy of Nature are divinely enriched with healing
powers for the mind and body."*
—DR. BACH

NORTH AMERICAN ESSENCES

*The various families of flower essences continue to be tested in hospitals,
clinics, and private practices throughout the world. The applications are
many and varied. These are a small sampling of some recorded studies.*

Three presentations of the findings of Dr. Jeffrey Cram, Ph.D.,
during the "2002 North American Flower Essence Society" training
session:

Study One:
Dr. Cram conducted double-blind studies with flower
essences using two FES formulas. In the first study, subjects
were exposed to an impossible arithmetic problem during
which time their muscle tension was studied. The outcome
found that flower essences appeared to help the participants
let go of distractions and foster a sense of calm, which
enabled them to concentrate on the math problem.

Study Two:

A researcher measured the brain waves in subjects under relaxed lighting conditions, then under the stress of harsh fluorescent lights. The first group received one of two different flower essence blends and the second group, a placebo. The group that received the flower essence blends had little reaction to the lights. The group that received the placebo experienced increased activity of the frontal lobes of the brain (the part of the brain responsible for the "fight or flight" syndrome). Dr. Cram concluded that the study may provide evidence of the ability of flower essences to strengthen emotional equilibrium and equanimity in the face of environmental stresses.

Study Three:

Dr. Cram used the Beck Depression Inventory and Hamilton Depression Scale to assess mild-to-moderately depressed individuals. Participants received a flower essence blend based on each client's personal issues (no two clients received the same essence blend). After one month, the depressive symptoms dropped 40%; after two months, there was a 50% drop. The reduction in depressive symptoms remained at 50% after a full three months.

"The smallest flower is a thought, a life answering to some feature of the Great Whole, of whom they have a persistent intuition."
–HONORE DE BALZAC

BACH FLOWER ESSENCES

This case study analysis indicated the potential of Bach flower essences as a means of pain relief. Among the 384 subjects studied, forty-one suffered from pain.

Their response to the therapy was surprising: 46% felt the treatment had relieved their pain. In 49% of the subjects, the physical outcome was unknown. The truly astounding finding was that 88% of all subjects, whether they suffered from pain or not, reported an improvement in their emotional outlook.

SWISS MEDICAL CHARITY - GREEN CROSS

The Australian combination flower remedy of *Electro Essence* was used to treat child victims from Belarus who were affected by the Chernobyl (Russian) nuclear disaster. They discovered that between one-third and one-half of the victims experienced a drop in radiation levels. Another ongoing trial is underway using the Australian Bush remedy *She Oak* for treating various hormonal issues.

HOSPITALS AND CLINICS
USING FLOWER ESSENCES

When you are admitted to a **Danish** hospital, you can choose to receive secondary treatment from a flower remedy practitioner as an additional treatment option.

Over sixteen hospitals throughout **Australia** currently offer flower essence treatments to their patients. Several clinics in western Australia that use flower essences in their drug and rehabilitation services found that, while 80% of heroin addicts relapsed quickly after treatment, the relapse rate was significantly reduced after using flower essences.

At the University of Sao Paulo in **Brazil,** Dr. Katia Kuchler used Australian Bush essences to treat diabetes. She discovered a significant reduction in glucose levels, pain, infection, and insomnia. In their burn unit the flower essence *Fireweed* is often used to promote healing.

Both the Cancer Care Center in Ft. Worth, **Texas,** and the Baylor Medical Center in Dallas have cancer support programs in which American *Petite Fleur* flower essences are given to help patients alleviate many of the adverse reactions to chemotherapy.

In **Japan,** the Niwa Clinic in Tokyo, and the Ando Clinic in Chiba-kin use flower essences in a variety of capacities.

LAR DO NENEN CHILDREN'S SHELTER

Suzana Loreto Maia (who has a degree in psychology with a specialization in psychomotricity) conducted a two-year study at *Lar Do Nenen*, a children's shelter in Recife, **Brazil**. The shelter looks after children from birth to two years old who have either been abandoned or are at risk.

Throughout the two-year period, Maia put flower essences in the children's bath, misted the air with essences, and used them in topical creams. In the beginning, she noticed small changes in their behavior, such as their ability to remain seated while looking at pictures in a book and an improvement in their overall behavior. A few weeks later, she noticed the children having fun organizing games among themselves, something she hadn't observed before.

The analysis of the data was compiled in two ways: the first group was studied throughout the entire period of use. The second group was studied for a beginning period, then again after a six-month period.

In conclusion, Maia observed that the children who had been taking flower essences for almost six months did not feel the need to sit on people's laps as much. They also showed an increased interest in learning games and in listening to music. Those who didn't take flower essences continued to show a lack of interest in learning and playing. Maia also observed that children who took flower essences generally fell ill less often and had fewer skin problems.

"He who lives in harmony with himself lives in harmony with the world."
–Marcus Aurelius

ITALIAN STUDIES

In Italy, Dr. S. Calzolari, a pediatrician, studied the effects of flower essences on 417 children with emotional difficulties. He concluded that they were very helpful and effective. Drs. D'Auria and Pezza also suggested that flower essences are especially effective in helping to control the psychological aspects of pain.

Another Italian study conducted in 1997 included 115 subjects who suffered from anxiety, depression, and stress. The subjects were treated with flower essences over a period of three and a half months.

The results showed positive improvement for 89% of the patients, especially those suffering from anxiety. Children and adolescents tended to respond more quickly to the treatment. Almost 95% of the subjects, who initially declared themselves skeptical about flower essence therapy, also enjoyed improvement in their conditions.

GERMAN STUDIES

A Hamburg psychiatrist and psychotherapist, Dr. Karin Hauffe, has long used flower essences for learning and behavioral problems in children. Dr. Hauffe also commented on the following situation: "I also use them [flower essences] for trauma and bad dreams. Recently, I saw a little boy who had been run over and was frightened of loud noises. After three days of treatment with the Australian Bush flower essences *Emergency Essence* and *Bush Fuchsia*, he was fine."

In 1996, a study was conducted at the University Hospital for Women in Heidelberg of twenty-four women in the first trimester of their pregnancies. Two professors, one from the Heidelberg University Hospital for Women and another from the Institute of Psychology in Tubingen, supervised the study. The twenty-four women were divided into three groups:

Group 1 received flower essences, *Group 2* received psychological counseling, and *Group 3* received "strict care" by an obstetrician. The results found that: *Group 1*, which used the flower essences, delivered infants with significantly less assistance than the "obstetrician control group." More significantly, the flower essence *Group 1* needed fewer drugs and exhibited less tension, decreased pain, and felt reduced levels of anxiety than did both *Group 2* and *Group 3*. It was concluded that the use of flower essences during pregnancy resulted in an easier delivery among the women studied.

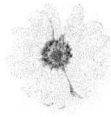

Chapter Nine
THE FLOWER ESSENCE KITCHEN

*"The discovery of a new dish does more for the
happiness of mankind than the discovery of a star."*
—ANTHELME BRILLAT-SAVARIN

FLOWER ESSENCE CAFÉ

Drawing on my years of experience as a cookbook author and columnist, I've assembled several recipes that incorporate, and are inspired by, flower essences. Eating these dishes will put a smile on anyone's face.

With this new twist on the "Alice B. Toklas" brownie, the challenge I faced in creating these recipes was to eliminate any heat element which would change the flower essence molecular structure.

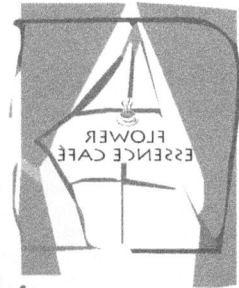

You can start your own *Flower Essence Café* by offering your friends and family dishes that incorporate the uplifting essence of flowers.

Enjoy!

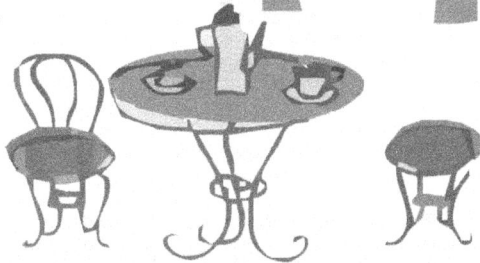

BAILEY TRANQUILITY POTATO SALAD
2 drops of Tranquility Mix Bailey Flower Essence Combination

8 unpeeled red potatoes. Bake until soft, then cube.

½ C peas, lightly steamed

½ C carrots, shredded

½ t ginger, freshly grated

1 t yellow whole grain mustard

1 t kosher salt

¼ - ½ C light mayonnaise
   (chipotle style [optional])

½ t smoky paprika

¼ C fresh parsley, cut small

2 T fresh chives, chopped small

PREPARATION
1. MIX ingredients together while potatoes are still warm, add essence.
2. CHILL at least one hour before serving.

"The chief pleasure in eating does not consist in costly seasoning or exquisite flavor, but in yourself."
–HORACE

HAPPY CALIFORNIAN CHAMOMILE GUACAMOLE WITH CORN-LIME CHIPS
4 drops of Chamomile flower essence

GUACAMOLE

1 large avocado

2 T lime juice

¼ t garlic powder, ¼ t cumin powder

½ t salt

1 red chili, whole dried, crushed

1 T canola oil

1 tomato, deseeded and cut into very small chunks

3 C corn chips, spread on a baking sheet. (Heat in medium oven for 2-3 minutes. Sprinkle with fresh lime juice just before serving.)

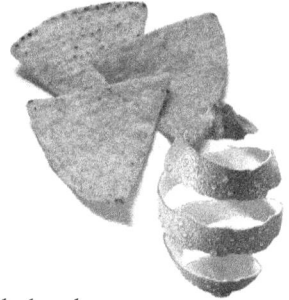

PREPARATION
1. MASH first five ingredients together using a fork.
2. ADD cut tomatoes and flower essence.
3. HEAT oil in a small pan then add chilies. Fry lightly until brown. Add to guacamole and mix together.
4. SERVE with warm corn-lime chips and prepared salsa.

CONTENTED HUMMUS LAVASH ROLL
5 drops of Black-Eyed Susan flower essence

3 medium garlic cloves (Cover with tin foil and roast in a 350 degree
oven for 30-45 minutes until soft.)
2 C canned chickpeas or cannelloni beans (rinse well and drain)
¼ C sesame paste (tahini), almond or sunflower butter
3 T olive oil
3 T freshly squeezed lemon juice
1 T lemon zest
1 t soy sauce or Braggs Liquid Aminos
1 t kosher or sea salt
½ t ground cumin, ¼ t ground coriander
¼ t smoky paprika
¼ t cayenne pepper
¼ C cold water, if needed
2 T fresh Italian parsley, minced
2 cucumbers, sliced paper thin using a mandolin
2 roasted red peppers, cut into thin slices
1 large whole wheat lavash bread

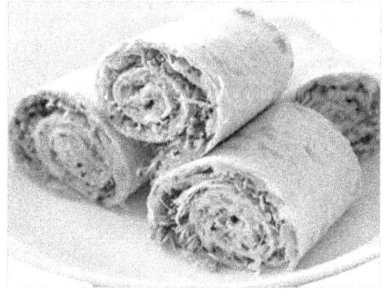

PREPARATION

1. PROCESS the roasted garlic cloves and rinsed beans in a food
   processor, pulse the machine a few times.
2. ADD tahini or nut butter, olive oil, lemon juice, zest, and soy
   sauce. Stop the processor occasionally to scrape down the sides
   of the bowl.
3. OPEN the lid and add the salt, cumin, coriander, paprika,
   cayenne, parsley, and flower essence. Process until thoroughly
   blended. If the puree seems too thick for spreading, pulse in up
   to ¼ cup of water.
4. TRANSFER the puree to a bowl. Cover with plastic wrap and
   refrigerate to chill well.
5. SPREAD hummus over entire bread. Top with one layer of
   cucumber and pepper slices and roll up tightly (on short side).
6. WRAP roll with plastic wrap and refrigerate for at least 1 hour.
7. CUT into 3-4" pieces just before serving.

HIMALAYAN PAKORA

These deep-fried fritters are a great snack any time of the day. They are served with coconut chutney (recipe next page).

2-2¼ C chickpea flour
2 T rice flour (optional)
½ t cumin seeds, toasted and slightly crushed
¼-½ t cayenne pepper or 1 freshly chopped Indian green chili, deseeded and chopped small
¼ t turmeric
½ t coriander powder
½ t ginger, freshly grated
1 T salt

1 cup water
1½ C vegetables, cut small (green pepper, onion, peas, eggplant, spinach, or cauliflower.)
¼ C cilantro leaves, chopped
½ t baking soda
Canola oil (for deep frying)

PREPARATION

1. MIX first eight ingredients together.
2. ADD water slowly to form a semi-thick, crepe-like batter, adjust water amount as needed.
3. ADD vegetables and cilantro leaves.
4. ADD baking soda just before frying.
5. HEAT oil to frying temperature, add 1 large spoonful of vegetable batter for each pakora. Fry until golden brown. Drain well on paper towels.
6. PREHEAT oven to 150 degrees. After fully draining on a paper towel, add to a baking dish placed in the preheated oven. This will keep the fried pakoras hot and fresh until the entire batch is cooked.

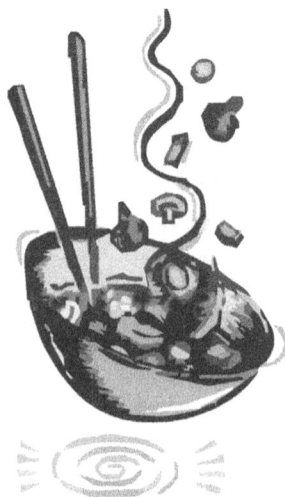

AWAKENED CHUTNEY
3 drops of Lotus flower essence

2 C mint or cilantro (coriander) leaves, fresh, or any combination
   of both
2 T tamarind paste or ⅛ C lemon juice
½ C unsweetened coconut, fresh or dry, grated
2" piece fresh ginger, either grated or cut into very small pieces
1 t brown sugar or Indian jaggery
1-2 green Indian or jalapeno chilies, fresh, or ½-1 t cayenne pepper
         (according to your heat index)
3 T pine nuts, peanuts, or macadamia nuts, toasted
1 t salt
⅛ - ¼ C water

SEASONING (optional)
*Heat the ghee or oil, then add mustard seeds until they pop. Add urad
dhal, stir until golden, add hing powder, then immediately take off heat.*
1 t *ghee* (clarified butter) or oil
½ t black mustard seeds
½ t urad dhal (available in an Indian grocery store)
Pinch of Asafoetida (hing) powder

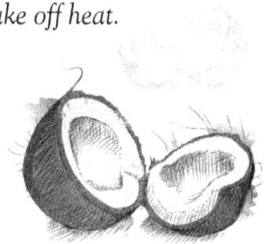

PREPARATION
1. CUT the green chilies and discard the seeds. Use them sparingly
    since they are quite powerful.
2. BLEND all ingredients, adjust water for a light sauce
    consistency.
3. ADD salt, adjust if needed; stir in seasoning and essence.

HOW TO MAKE CLARIFIED BUTTER (GHEE)
*In a heavy-duty pot, bring one pound of sweet butter to a gentle boil. Lower the heat so that
butter continues to boil very slowly. Leave it on the stove about half an hour until the fat
has separated from the butter and liquid has become clear. At this point, the fat can burn
quickly so make sure to check it often. Let ghee cool, scrap-off top layer, and strain through
a layered cheese cloth into a clean, completely dry jar. It can remain fresh for many months
as long as no moisture gets in the jar.*

CALMING SMOKED SALMON PINWHEELS
2 drops of Valerian flower essence

1 C reduced, nonfat, or vegan cream cheese, bring to room temperature
2 T chopped fresh dill, or 1 t dried dill
4 whole wheat flour tortillas (10")
1 C smoked salmon (lox), finely chopped
16 fresh baby spinach leaves
1 roasted yellow bell pepper. Cool, then cut into very thin strips (16 pieces)

PREPARATION

1. MIX flower essence in softened cream cheese and add dill.
2. SPREAD about ¼ C cream cheese mixture over each tortilla.
3. SPRINKLE each tortilla with ¼ C chopped lox.
3. PLACE 4 spinach leaves and 4 bell pepper strips on each tortilla.
4. ROLL up tortillas tightly. Spread a little cream cheese mixture to seal roll. Wrap securely with plastic wrap. Refrigerate at least 2 hours, but no longer than 24 hours.
5. SERVE by cutting tortilla rolls into 1-inch pieces. Place cut side up on a serving platter.

FROSTING FOR SCONES
¼ cup powdered sugar, sifted. 1 T freshly squeezed lemon juice. 1 t lemon zest ½ t lavender. Add flower essence drops to frosting. Adjust thickness of frosting by adding a few drops of water until it is a drizzle consistency.

LEMONY-LAVENDER SERENITY SCONES
2 drops of Gentian flower essence

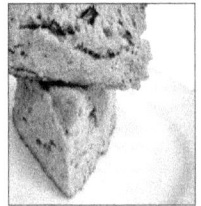

2 C unbleached organic white flour
1½ t salt, 1 t baking powder, 1 t baking soda
⅓ C natural brown granulated or maple sugar
Finely grated zest of 2 lemons
2 t finely chopped lavender, dried, cooking grade
    (Save ½ t lavender for the frosting)
½ C unsalted butter or margarine, chilled and cubed
¾ C vanilla low or nonfat yogurt
2 eggs, beaten until fluffy

PREPARATION

1. PREHEAT oven to 400 degrees. Line a baking sheet with parchment paper and set aside.
2. SIFT flour, salt, baking powder, and baking soda into bowl. Add sugar, lemon zest, and 1½ t of the lavender.
3. ADD chilled butter or margarine and work it into flour ingredients until butter pieces are the size of small peas.
4. COMBINE yogurt and eggs and add to dry ingredients. Stir in just enough so it forms a dough.
5. KNEAD dough lightly, folding and flattening it several times.
6. PAT dough into a 6-inch circle, approximately 1-inch thick. Transfer onto prepared baking sheet. Brush top with 1 t yogurt. Sprinkle 1 t sugar over the top. Score circle into eight wedges, cutting almost to bottom.
7. BAKE 23-25 minutes until golden brown. Cool on baking sheet.
8. MAKE a thin frosting by combining ½ t lavender with powered sugar, lemon juice, and essence.
9. CUT scones into wedges. Drizzle icing over cooled scones.

FRUIT SALAD WITH ROSE DRESSING
2 drops of Neem flower essence

6 C any combination of fruits, cut into small, bite-size pieces.
2 T lemon juice, freshly squeezed

DRESSING
2 C low or nonfat vanilla yogurt
1 t cardamom powder
2 drops pure rosewater (available in Indian grocery stores)

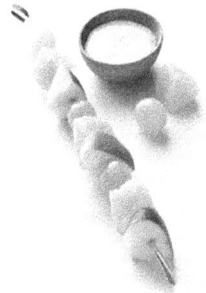

PREPARATION

1. ADD lemon juice to fruit, skewer 7-8 pieces and chill.
2. WHIP dressing with flower essence until very light and airy.
3. SERVE by arranging skewers on a large platter. Serve dressing on the side in individual small bowls.

AUSTRALIAN WATTLE ROCKY ROAD DARK CHOCOLATE CRACKIES
5 drops of Sunshine Wattle flower essence

Chocolate crackies are a favorite of Australian children and are often served at parties.

CRACKIES
Makes about 24 pieces
1 C powdered sugar
½ C dark cocoa powder
4 C crispy rice cereal (brown rice cereal is a good alternative)
1 C unsweetened coconut, dried, shredded
¾ C butter or margarine, melted

TOPPING
½ C any dried fruit (I use pineapple) roughly chopped small. (You can use cooking shears coated with a drop of oil to cut the fruit.)
½ C pecans or walnuts, dry toasted, chopped very small

PREPARATION
1. SIFT together the powdered sugar and cocoa powder into a large bowl. Stir in the crispy rice and dried coconut.
2. MELT butter or margarine over low flame. Stir in dry ingredients until well-mixed.
3. SCOOP crackie mix into paper muffin cups.
4. MIX topping mixture together with flower essence.
5. TOP with 1 T of topping and press into mixture.
6. CHILL in the fridge until firm.

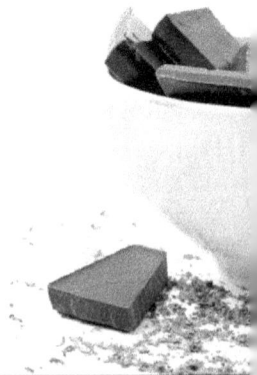

HEART CENTERED ROSE - TEAKWOOD LASSIE DRINK

4 Cups

3 drops of Teakwood Flower flower essence

4 C low or nonfat plain yogurt
5 T lavender, or any mild honey or agave syrup
2 drops pure rosewater
(available in an Indian grocery store)
½ t fresh cardamom powder
2 C ice, roughly chopped

PREPARATION
1. WHIP first four ingredients together in a blender with flower essence, blend until well-mixed.
2. ADD ½ C ice to glass, fill with yogurt mixture.

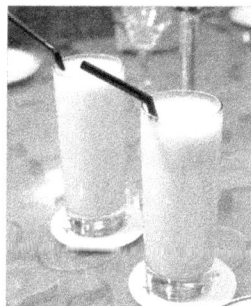

CALIFORNIA ORANGE/MANGO MORNING GLORY PUNCH

4 Glasses

2 drops of Morning Glory flower essence

4 C orange juice
1 C mango pulp
1 C raspberry spritzer

½ orange, cut into thin slices, remove seeds
¼ C raspberries, fresh
8 mint leaves

PREPARATION
1. BLEND juice, pulp, spritzer, and flower essence together.
2. ADD 1 C of punch to each stemmed glass.
3. TOP with orange slice, a few raspberries, and mint leaves.

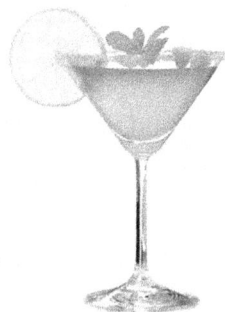

4 Bowls

CHETANA'S REFRESHING CHILLED CANTALOUPE SOUP

2 drops of Almond flower essence

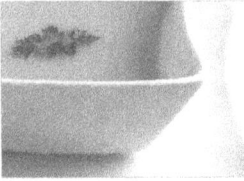

1 cantaloupe, chopped
2 C orange juice
½ t ginger powder
¼ t nutmeg, freshly grated
½ t salt
pinch of chipotle pepper or cayenne powder

GARNISH
1 T fennel fronds, top of the fennel bulb, chopped

PREPARATION
1. BLEND six ingredients together with flower essence until well-mixed, chill.
2. TOP with fronds.

"Cookery means the knowledge of all herbs, fruits, balms, and spices, and all that is healing and sweet in the fields and groves. It means carefulness, inventiveness, willingness, and readiness of appliances. It means the economy of your grandmothers and the science of the modern chemist; it means much testing and no wasting."
—JOHN RUSKIN
(Quoted in the first edition of the
Boston Cooking-School Cook Book, 1896)

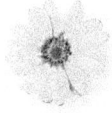

Chapter Ten

CONCLUSION

"The Earth laughs in flowers."
—Ralph Waldo Emerson

AWE-INSPIRING POSSIBILITIES

E ven though Dr. Edward Bach spent the last half of his life dedicated to researching flower essences and making them widely accessible, just before his death he deliberately destroyed his developmental research notes and many of his writings. He wanted to ensure that there would be no misinterpretation of his research after he died. What he left behind was a foundation of thirty-eight essences developed as a "whole person" healing system. Because of Dr. Bach's pioneering work, it is now relatively easy to find Bach Flower Essences on pharmacy and natural food store shelves throughout the world! The works of other leading flower essence pioneers, several of whom are featured in this book, are also quickly finding their way into the mainstream of American complementary health care. These flower essence families have already become firmly established in their native cultures and lands of origin. How fortunate we are that

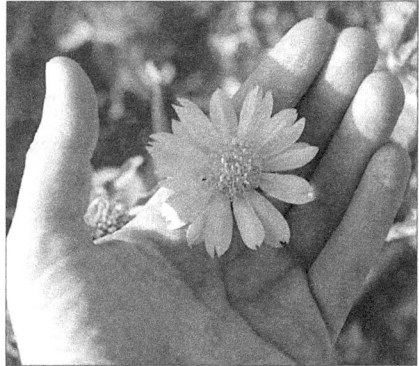

these powerful healing properties—this "liquid energy" inherent in flowers—has been re-discovered.

Our modern lives are no longer in tune with the seasons of nature as were previous generations and the digital age we live in is producing a generation alienated and isolated. The outcome of this is that the stresses of daily living bombards us much too fast, which can create an atmosphere of imbalance and ill health. Unfortunately, the remedies and pharmaceuticals we rely on to mitigate our disease are so strong that the side effects often do more harm than good. So when we open ourselves up to the energetic, vibrational aspects of flower essences, which have been with us through the centuries, they offer an ideal balm for these times.

"We are all inventors, each sailing out on a voyage of discovery, guided each by a private chart, of which there is no duplicate. The world is all gates, all opportunities."
–Ralph Waldo Emerson

These pages share the absolute beauty of flower essences and how they can help us return to our natural state of balance. And flower essences are all about "balance." An example of this is someone who wears two shoes of different heights; the outcome may be that a leg or shoulder begins to ache. Being out of balance, in body, mind, or spirit, can often create new, unrelated problems. "Being in balance" also means that we experience the harmony and well-being of our natural state of wholeness—a subtle integrated alignment where vibrant health is our birthright. Without this re-alignment, life can be burdensome; it's like being on a train and holding the luggage on our laps when we can just as easily put the luggage down and enjoy the ride.

My heartfelt intent in writing this book is to instill some of the wonder and efficacy that I have found these gifts of nature to possess. We have traveled this journey of exploration together through the fascinating history of flower essences, the unique diagnostic approach, and their practical application in our lives. My hope is that you, too, may become inspired to open yourself to the awe-inspiring and healing possibilities inherent in the humble yet majestic flower.

REFERENCE MATERIALS

Books

Some of these books may only be available online since they are produced outside of the United States. www.Amazon.com is always a good starting point if you would like to purchase some reference material.

The Bach Flower Remedies
By Edward Bach
This is a great introductory book. It begins with Dr. Bach's initial writings on flower remedies, which were published under the name, *Heal Thyself.* The book provides detailed descriptions of each essence and an overview of the various emotional states they address.

The Medical Discoveries of Edward Bach
By Nora Weeks
This fascinating biography of Dr. Bach is written by one of his closest associates. It presents the dramatic story of his life, work, and discoveries. The story chronicles Bach's struggles and his ultimate success in bringing flower essences into wide acceptance in the modern world.

Bach Flower Remedies for Children
By Barbara Mazzarella
This book is designed for parents to help them find the right flower remedy for their children. The use of each essence is summarized through a fairy tale, which helps to highlight the issue related to the remedy and its healing abilities. Each selection also ends with a poem.

Bach Flower Therapy, Theory and Practice
By Mechthild Scheffer
Each Bach flower remedy is explored in detail starting with its botanical attributes, the principles of the remedy, key symptoms for taking the remedy, energy block symptoms, potential results, supportive aspects, and a positive statement.

Advanced Bach Flower Therapy
By Gotz Blome, M.D.
This is an excellent reference book. It is an exhaustive resource for those who know the fundamentals of flower essence therapy but would like a more in-depth look at treatment options.

Treating Animal Illnesses & Emotional States with Flower Essence Remedies
By Jessica Bear, Ph.D., N.D. and Tricia Lewis
This is one of the more comprehensive books on treating animals with Bach and other flower remedy groups. It offers guidance on selecting a remedy based on the emotional state of the animal and its personality type.

Australian Bush Flower Essences
By Ian White
This is a comprehensive book by the founder of Australian Bush flower essences. This book reveals the physical attributes of each essence, the lore and history, plus its healing properties. Each essence is covered in detail indicating both the negative condition and positive outcome.

The Essence of Healing: A Guide to the Alaskan Flower, Gem, and Environmental Essences
By Steve Johnson
This unique collection of flower, gem, and environmental essences from the wilderness areas of Alaska is the result of more than twelve years of research in both field and therapeutic settings. The book contains very useful information on how to select and use the Alaskan family of flower essences.

Flower Essence Repertory
By Patricia Kaminski
This book features the selections of California flower essences from one of the Flower Essence Society (FES) founders. It is clear and informative, easy to use, and serves as a helpful guidebook.

The New Encyclopedia of Flower Remedies
By Clare G. Harvey
This is one of most comprehensive books on the worldwide groups of flower essences. It combines the properties, insight, history, and reasons to use specific essences and is written by one of the most well-known complementary therapists and authorities on flower essences.

Heal Yourself with Flowers and Other Essences
By Nikki Bradford
This is a very informative book that includes lovely color photography. It highlights 150 essences from around the world, describes their healing components and properties, and indicates their use and beneficial affects.

Vibrational Medicine: The #1 Handbook of Subtle-Energy Therapies
By Richard Gerber
Dr. Gerber provides an encyclopedic understanding of vibrational healing therapy, a comprehensive approach which may be a bit dense for someone new to flower essences. If you wish to dive deep into the theory and practice of complementary healing systems, Dr. Gerber's book is a very useful tool.

Online Resources
General Flower Essences (21 families): www.essencesonline.com
Bach Flower Essence Information: www.bachcentre.com
Discounted Bach Flower Essences: www.swansonvitamins.com
Australian Bush Essences: www.ausflowers.com.au
Alaskan Flower Essences: www.alaskanessences.com
Flower Essence Society: www.fesflowers.com
Bailey Essences: www.baileyessences.com
Himalayan Essences: www.aumhimalaya.com

If you are interested in purchasing *Flower Essences Healing Crèmes*, or contacting Joan Greenblatt, please visit:
www.EssentialFlowerRemedies.com

Selections from five flower essence families, aromatherapeutic extracts, along with the 38 Bach essences, are listed here. To obtain a complete list or purchase specific essences, refer to the books and web links provided on the previous pages.

HIMALAYAN FLOWER ESSENCES

ASHOKA FLOWER: *Saraca indica*
KEY ASPECT: DEEP SORROW
PATTERNS OF IMBALANCE: Deep-seated sadness, grief, and disharmony of one's inner being; may be due to events such as: bereavement, failure, suffering, disease, or isolation.
POSITIVE QUALITIES: Produces a profound inner state of joy, harmony, and well-being. Beneficial for the elderly and helpful for infertile women.

LOTUS: *Nelumbo nucifera*
KEY ASPECT: SPIRITUALLY DEPLETED
PATTERNS OF IMBALANCE: Restlessness during meditation; lack of concentration; disconnected from spiritual self.
POSITIVE QUALITIES: Allows for a gentle release of emotions; hastens recovery from illness; aids healers in diagnosing their patients' conditions more accurately; a spiritual elixir.

NEEM: *Azadirchta indica*
KEY ASPECT: OVERLY INTELLECTUAL
PATTERNS OF IMBALANCE: Overly cerebral people who are not centered within themselves.
POSITIVE QUALITIES: Helps bring love, empathy, intuition, and a less judgmental attitude.

PARROT TREE FLOWER: *Butea monosperma*
KEY ASPECT: PUBLIC EXPRESSION
PATTERNS OF IMBALANCE: Public speakers who need to improve the timing of their elocution; challenges in coordinating thought and speech.
POSITIVE QUALITIES: Helps improve and enhance pronunciation, enunciation, and vocal expression; promotes self-confidence in public speaking.

PEACOCK FLOWER: *Poinciana pulcherrima*
K EY A SPECT : A DDICTIVE B EHAVIOR
PATTERNS OF IMBALANCE: Rehabilitation challenges, specifically regarding treatment of drug addicts; imbalance due to long debilitating illness.
POSITIVE QUALITIES: Restores sensitivity of the nervous system; eases physical and mental torture.

TEAKWOOD FLOWER: *Tectona grandis*
K EY A SPECT : E LDERLY I SSUES
PATTERNS OF IMBALANCE: Senile dementia, irrationality, confusion, and tiredness of old age.
POSITIVE QUALITIES: A vitalizing, refreshing essence for anyone over sixty years; enhances the ability to concentrate, communicate, and keep the mind interested and vital.

BAILEY ESSENCES

ALMOND: *Prunus dulcis*
K EY A SPECT : D ISCONNECTED WITH I NNER S ELF
PATTERNS OF IMBALANCE: Entanglement in past difficulties, old patterns; unable to see the road ahead; out of alignment with one's inner spirit.
POSITIVE QUALITIES: Helps the re-establishment of one's supportive inner guide; renews the sense of connectedness with the soul; encourages intuition, understanding of past patterns and life lessons.

BISTORT: *Polygonum bistorta*
K EY A SPECT : D EALING WITH C HANGE
PATTERNS OF IMBALANCE: During times of transition resulting in negativity and depression; stuck in old ways; feeling threatened and vulnerable due to life changes.
POSITIVE QUALITIES: An inner scaffold to maintain the basic structure of one's personality and provide loving support during life changes; converts a possible breakdown into a breakthrough.

FUJI CHERRY: *Prunus incisa*
KEY ASPECT: BODILY TENSION
PATTERNS OF IMBALANCE: When the mind is tense creating stress in the body; for times when one becomes overly caught up in life issues.
POSITIVE QUALITIES: Encourages relaxation; to help look at life calmly and with more detachment; to let go. A soothing essence for developing a quiet reflective and tranquil mind.

HEATH BEDSTRAW: *Galium saxatile*
KEY ASPECT: RESTLESSNESS AND HOLDING ON
PATTERNS OF IMBALANCE: Inner restlessness; holding on to concepts and beliefs.
POSITIVE QUALITIES: Helps one return to inner stillness and the peace of a tranquil state; combines well with other essences that promote letting go and transitioning through change.

ORIENTAL POPPY: *Papaver somniferum*
KEY ASPECT: DEPENDENCY ISSUES
PATTERNS OF IMBALANCE: Sleep-walking through dependant situations; debilitating dependency on a substance, person, or situation.
POSITIVE QUALITIES: Helps one to wake up and energetically change one's life; releases and balances obsessive and co-dependent behavior.

SOLOMON'S SEAL: *Polygonatum verticillatum*
KEY ASPECT: BUSY MIND
PATTERNS OF IMBALANCE: An overly "busy" person who never seems to finish things; bogged down in trivia; the chattering mind.
POSITIVE QUALITIES: Helps one reassert control over a wayward mind and an overly busy life; ability to fulfill one's own needs and not be exploited by others.

WHITE DEAD NETTLE: *Lamium album*
KEY ASPECT: REVOLVING THOUGHT PATTERNS
PATTERNS OF IMBALANCE: Thought patterns that keep revolving and will not stop; "hamster on the treadmill" syndrome; addicted to objects, events, or people; OCD (obsessive compulsive disorder).
POSITIVE QUALITIES: Eliminates the tiring effects of obsessive thought patterns; helps one to detach from emotional addiction.

BACH FLOWER ESSENCES

AGRIMONY: *Agrimonia eupatoria*
KEY ASPECT: HIDDEN ANXIETY
PATTERNS OF IMBALANCE: Hides troubles and anxieties behind a smiling face; makes light of inner difficulties; rarely burdens others; avoids arguments and confrontations; may lead to alcohol or drugs.
POSITIVE QUALITIES: Helps to acknowledge and transcend dishonest feelings; enhances one's ability to truly expose and express oneself.

ASPEN: *Populus tremula*
KEY ASPECT: FEAR OF UNKNOWN THINGS
PATTERNS OF IMBALANCE: Vague, irrational, troubling fears and anxieties, sudden apprehension; may take the form of nightmares; could be related to religious or spiritual beliefs and concepts.
POSITIVE QUALITIES: Promotes courage in exploring the unknown and trust issues; release of shadow-like fears.

BEECH: *Fagus sylvatica*
KEY ASPECT: JUDGEMENTAL
PATTERNS OF IMBALANCE: Intolerance, overly critical, finds fault with others. Tension which often affects the upper chest, jaws, and hands.
POSITIVE QUALITIES: Helps bring compassion, non-judgement, empathy, and acceptance of other peoples' differences.

CENTAURY: *Centaurium umbellatum*
KEY ASPECT: WEAK PERSONALITY
PATTERNS OF IMBALANCE: Too timid, with an excessive desire to please others; difficulty in saying "no," even when exploited; overextends oneself; often affects the shoulders and back.
POSITIVE QUALITIES: Promotes strength and courage to fearlessly follow one's own true path and stand up for oneself; self-determination; acting decisively.

CERATO: *Ceratostigma willmottiana*
KEY ASPECT: LACK OF SELF-TRUST
PATTERNS OF IMBALANCE: Not trusting the wisdom of one's own judgment; always seeks approval and asks advice and opinions of others; easily led astray.
POSITIVE QUALITIES: Promotes trust and confidence in one's inner sense of knowing.

CHERRY PLUM: *Prunus cerasifera*
KEY ASPECT: LOSING CONTROL
PATTERNS OF IMBALANCE: Fear of losing control of one's thoughts and actions; doing things one knows may be wrong; effects of prolonged warfare; trauma from a series of profound life events.
POSITIVE QUALITIES: Promotes release of one's irrational impulses; empowers one to learn positive lessons from frightening events in one's life.

CHESTNUT BUD: *Ceratostigma willmottiana*
KEY ASPECT: NOT LEARNING LESSONS
PATTERNS OF IMBALANCE: Repeats the same mistakes over and over again; slow to learn from past experience; careless, clumsy, and inattentive.
POSITIVE QUALITIES: Helps one to become a good learner and pay attention to what's happening in the present; helps one formulate wise responses from lessons learned.

CHICORY: *Chichorium intybus*
KEY ASPECT: POSSESSIVE LOVE
PATTERNS OF IMBALANCE: Overly involved with and possessive of family and close friends; imposes one's own standards on loved ones; bossy, selfish, demands attention.
POSITIVE QUALITIES: Promotes unconditional love for those in one's life without smothering them.

CLEMATIS: *Clematis vitalba*
KEY ASPECT: DREAMING INDIFFERENCE
PATTERNS OF IMBALANCE: Daydreamer, absentminded, withdraws into fantasy worlds; ungrounded and indifferent to the details of everyday life; prone to drowsiness, excessive sleepiness.
POSITIVE QUALITIES: Promotes an established bridge between the physical world and the world of ideas; helps to become awake and alive to the present moment.

CRAB APPLE: *Malus pumila*
KEY ASPECT: CLEANSING REMEDY
PATTERNS OF IMBALANCE: Shame, feeling of uncleanliness; poor image of one's personal self and the environment; obsessed by trivial matters.
POSITIVE QUALITIES: This essence teaches acceptance of the body and the environment on all levels—physical, emotional, and spiritual.

ELM: *Ulmus procera*
KEY ASPECT: TEMPORARILY OVERWHELMED
PATTERNS OF IMBALANCE: Overburdened by responsibilities; for the occasional feeling that a task is just too difficult or that one is inadequate to accomplish it.
POSITIVE QUALITIES: Promotes composure and a return of one's natural ability to handle responsibility with ease.

GENTIAN: *Gentiana amarella*
KEY ASPECT: DAY-TO-DAY DISCOURAGEMENTS
PATTERNS OF IMBALANCE: Feelings of discouragement, depression, sadness, or doubt, which may be caused by even small day-to-day obstacles.
POSITIVE QUALITIES: Promotes confidence and perseverance to help overcome one's daily challenges.

GORSE: *Ulex europaeus*
KEY ASPECT: RELENTLESS DESPAIR
PATTERNS OF IMBALANCE: Great hopelessness and despair; life seems a misery; gives up and believes that nothing more can be done; often present in the case of chronic illness.
POSITIVE QUALITIES: Promotes confidence in obtaining a solution or possibility; helps one to "see light at the end of the tunnel," which is an important component of healing.

HEATHER: *Calluna vulgaris*
KEY ASPECT: SELF-CENTEREDNESS
PATTERNS OF IMBALANCE: Constant talkers, especially about themselves and their problems; self-absorbed, greedy for other's attention; energy sapper; dislikes being alone.
POSITIVE QUALITIES: Promotes the ability to be open, listen sensitively with true empathy for others.

HOLLY: *Ilex aquifolium*
KEY ASPECT: EXTREME NEGATIVITY
PATTERNS OF IMBALANCE: Troubled by feelings of envy, suspicion, revenge, or hatred; disconnected from one's own source of love; feels that the love of others can't be trusted.
POSITIVE QUALITIES: Promotes unconditional love and goodwill; opens the heart to the full flow of love; helps one express the positive aspects of one's feelings.

HONEYSUCKLE: *Lonicera caprifolium*
KEY ASPECT: ABSORBED IN PAST
PATTERNS OF IMBALANCE: Nostalgia; dwells too much in the past, especially on loved ones, grief, or on ambitions that were never realized; often tinged with a feeling of pessimism.
POSITIVE QUALITIES: To learn from the past as a way to live joyfully and fully in the present.

HORNBEAM: *Carpinus betulus*
KEY ASPECT: MONDAY MORNING BLUES
PATTERNS OF IMBALANCE: Temporarily overwhelmed, bored, lack of energy; occurs often upon waking when one doesn't have strength to get through the routines of the day; convalescents.
POSITIVE QUALITIES: Restores mental liveliness and alertness; promotes enthusiasm to wake up each morning to a joyous and inspired life.

IMPATIENS: *Impatiens glandulifera*
KEY ASPECT: IMPATIENCE AND ANNOYANCE
PATTERNS OF IMBALANCE: Acts and thinks quickly; irritable at hindrances, impulsive, annoyed by hesitation or delay; intolerant of the slowness of others; pent-up tension and indigestion.
POSITIVE QUALITIES: Promotes empathy, understanding, patience in oneself and others; greater patience in dealing with life experiences and events.

LARCH: *Larix decidua*
KEY ASPECT: NEGATIVE PROGRAMMING
PATTERNS OF IMBALANCE: Lack of self-confidence; passive, hesitant; trapped in self-doubt; sense of inferiority; anticipates failure, often making no attempt to succeed; false modesty.
POSITIVE QUALITIES: Promotes courage, self-confidence, and determination to take on what one perceives to be ones challenges; clears old patterns of limitation.

MIMULUS: *Mimulus guttatus*
KEY ASPECT: KNOWN FEARS
PATTERNS OF IMBALANCE: Known fears of the dark, heights, water, disease, spiders, flying, death, poverty, etc.; also for extreme shyness.
POSITIVE QUALITIES: Promotes freedom from fear and anxiety.

MUSTARD: *Sinapis arvensis*
KEY ASPECT: SUDDEN GLOOM
PATTERNS OF IMBALANCE: Depression due to unknown cause; a sudden gloom which descends for no apparent reason; deep sadness and melancholy.
POSITIVE QUALITIES: Promotes peace, inner stability, cheerfulness, and serenity.

OAK: *Quercus robur*
KEY ASPECT: OVER EXTENDER
PATTERNS OF IMBALANCE: Overly responsible; plodder; battles on mindlessly when exhausted; depressed by chronic overwork.
POSITIVE QUALITIES: Brings joy and balance into one's endeavors; revives energy and allows one to enjoy a break from self-imposed hard work.

OLIVE: *Olea europaea*
KEY ASPECT: EXTREME EXHAUSTION
PATTERNS OF IMBALANCE: Mental and physical exhaustion, especially when caused by a long or debilitating illness; personal ordeals such as divorce, bankruptcy, or intense conflict.
POSITIVE QUALITIES: Assists in renewal; refreshes the spirit, gives strength and vitality.

PINE: *Pinus sylvestris*
KEY ASPECT: GUILT AND BLAME
PATTERNS OF IMBALANCE: Never satisfied; suffers from feelings of guilt, blame, and self-reproach; blames oneself for others' mistakes.
POSITIVE QUALITIES: Promotes self-acceptance, freedom from guilt, blame, and regret.

RED CHESTNUT: *Aesculus carnea*
KEY ASPECT: FEAR FOR LOVED ONE'S WELFARE
PATTERNS OF IMBALANCE: Over concern, worry, and fear for the welfare of loved ones; apprehension that terrible things may happen to them; projects anxiety onto loved ones; imagines the worst.
POSITIVE QUALITIES: Promotes expression of positive thoughts; letting go and release of anxious feeling toward loved ones; brings trust and confidence in the ability of others to look after themselves.

ROCK ROSE: *Helianthemum nummularium*
KEY ASPECT: EXTREME FRIGHT
PATTERNS OF IMBALANCE: All cases of extreme fear; paralysed by terror, panic, or urgency; trembling.
POSITIVE QUALITIES: Calmly faces challenging or transforming events, which result in an appropriate response. Soothing effect for panic attacks.

ROCK WATER
KEY ASPECT: EXTREMIST
PATTERNS OF IMBALANCE: Excessively hard on oneself; often adopts repressive or rigid personal regimes; dogmatic; spiritual pride; denies oneself.
POSITIVE QUALITIES: Facilitates a flexible aptitude and open-mindedness; helps promote balance and harmony in relationships and with the natural order of things.

SCLERANTHUS: *Scleranthus annuus*
KEY ASPECT: INABILITY TO CHOOSE
PATTERNS OF IMBALANCE: Torn between choices and can't decide between them; procrastination and uncertainty; mood swings; lack of concentration, restlessness, and indecision.
POSITIVE QUALITIES: Brings concentration, decisiveness, and stability; integration of emotional and intellectual extremes.

STAR OF BETHLEHEM: *Ornithogalum umbellatum*
KEY ASPECT: GREAT SHOCK
PATTERNS OF IMBALANCE: Trauma from the shock of bad news, of loss, an accident, or even birth; for traumatic events, whether experienced recently or in the past.
POSITIVE QUALITIES: Deeply restorative and soothing properties for shock or trauma. Helps acknowledge and transcend trauma; release of residual blocks, especially from the past; establishes equilibrium and comfort.

SWEET CHESTNUT: *Castanea sativa*
KEY ASPECT: MENTAL ANGUISH
PATTERNS OF IMBALANCE: Extreme anguish; reaching the limits of one's endurance, that the mind and body will give way; "the dark night of the soul."
POSITIVE QUALITIES: Creates a "life tether," a hidden reserve when trauma occurs; restores trust in oneself and the benevolence of the universe; helps the return of one's strength and sense of hope.

VERVAIN: *Verbena officinalis*
KEY ASPECT: RIGID VIEWS
PATTERNS OF IMBALANCE: Need to convince others of the correctness of personal beliefs; when excessive fervor and enthusiasm causes exhaustion; often associated with a missionary type of zeal.
POSITIVE QUALITIES: Allows one to see other viewpoints; imparts a genuine empathy; helps one to become an example that encourages and inspires others.

VINE: *Vitis vinifera*
KEY ASPECT: INFLEXIBILITY AND DOMINANCE
PATTERNS OF IMBALANCE: Insists that others do things their way; the "bully," "boss," or "dictator" personality; feels the need to control others.
POSITIVE QUALITIES: Teaches respect for other people's leadership; helps one discover and respect positive qualities in others; fosters a sense of compassion.

WALNUT: *Juglans regia*
KEY ASPECT: CHANGE AND UNWANTED INFLUENCE
PATTERNS OF IMBALANCE: Problems dealing with outside forces; to help move on and break old links and patterns; on the brink of major change such as divorce, puberty, menopause, or change in residence.
POSITIVE QUALITIES: Helps to ease transition; allows one to break free from outside influences and others' strong opinions. (A good essence for therapists to spray in their offices.)

WATER VIOLET: *Hottonia palustris*
KEY ASPECT: PRIDE AND ALOOFNESS
PATTERNS OF IMBALANCE: Overly self-reliant; loners who retreat and isolate themselves; can be proud and aloof; stiffness, and rigidity; prone to physical tension.
POSITIVE QUALITIES: Allows for communication and the ability to ask for help when needed; shares with others without sacrificing one's independence.

WHITE CHESTNUT: *Aesculus hippocastanum*
KEY ASPECT: PERSISTENT THOUGHTS
PATTERNS OF IMBALANCE: Unwanted thoughts; worries, ideas, or mental arguments, revolving endlessly; may cause insomnia and headaches.
POSITIVE QUALITIES: Quiets and calms the mental process; helps the mind to function clearly and effectively; fosters peace and contentment within.

WILD OAT: *Bromus ramosus*
KEY ASPECT: VOCATIONAL INDECISION
PATTERNS OF IMBALANCE: Unfulfilled ambition; unable to find direction in one's career; no clear sense of purpose; feels dissatisfied, uncertain, and bored with present situation.
POSITIVE QUALITIES: Helps one tune into one's inner self and find meaning and focus; clarifies direction, especially regarding one's life vocation and calling.

WILD ROSE: *Rosa canina*
KEY ASPECT: UNMOTIVATED AND APATHETIC
PATTERNS OF IMBALANCE: Resignation and apathy; fatalistic; lacks vitality; feels dull.
POSITIVE QUALITIES: Fosters motivation, creativity, and enthusiasm; re-energizes the dynamic quality in one's life.

WILLOW: *Salix vitellina*
KEY ASPECT: SELF-PITY AND RESENTMENT
PATTERNS OF IMBALANCE: Resentment; the persistent feeling that life is unfair; one may also resent the cheerfulness of others and bear grudges; can bring on arthritic conditions.
POSITIVE QUALITIES: Teaches one to take responsibility for one's own life, without pity or embitterment; creates optimism and a happy disposition.

RESCUE REMEDY: *Rock Rose, Cherry Plum, Clematis, Impatiens, and Star of Bethlehem.*
KEY ASPECT: EMERGENCIES
PATTERNS OF IMBALANCE: Emergency situations, shock, unconsciousness, emotional or physical stress.
POSITIVE QUALITIES: Helps to stabilize one's emotions during life trials. Restores a sense of balance when experiencing shock or trauma. (Can be taken up to five minutes apart until situation is stabilized.)

BLACK SPRUCE: *Picea mariana*
KEY ASPECT: OUT OF TOUCH WITH THE PRESENT
PATTERNS OF IMBALANCE: Contracted view of life; tendency to forget information learned from past experience; out of touch with the wisdom of one's soul.
POSITIVE QUALITIES: Supports the integration of past lessons and experiences into present time awareness; helps one draw inspiration from the wisdom of the ages.

FOXGLOVE: *Digitalis purpurea*
KEY ASPECT: LOSS OF PERSPECTIVE
PATTERNS OF IMBALANCE: Fear of the unknown; lack of perspective on how to deal with a challenging situation; unable to see the lesson or issue at the heart of a conflict or difficulty.
POSITIVE QUALITIES: Stimulates the release of fear and emotional tension; enables one's perception to expand to connect with the truth of a situation.

LAMB'S QUARTER: *Chenopodium album*
KEY ASPECT: LACK OF INTEGRATION
PATTERNS OF IMBALANCE: Lack of balance and harmony between mind and heart, the rational and the intuitive.
POSITIVE QUALITIES: Heals separation; balances the power of the mind with the joy of the heart.

MONKSHOOD: *Aconitum delphinifolium*
KEY ASPECT: SPIRITUAL IDENTITY AND CONFUSION
PATTERNS OF IMBALANCE: Difficulty experiencing close physical contact with others; confused sense of spiritual identity; lack of will in defining boundaries.
POSITIVE QUALITIES: Provides protection and support within the deepest levels of one's self; strengthen's personal interaction; fosters inner clarity.

OPIUM POPPY: *Papaver Sominifera*
KEY ASPECT: UNABLE TO INTEGRATE LEARNED LESSONS
PATTERNS OF IMBALANCE: Unable to find balance between activity and rest; deep exhaustion; unappreciative of past accomplishments; difficulty understanding and integrating life lessons and experiences.
POSITIVE QUALITIES: Helps one find a balance between doing and being; clears deep exhaustion; allows one to integrate and learn from previous experience.

VALERIAN: *Valeriana officinalis*
KEY ASPECT: INHARMONIOUS RELATIONSHIPS
PATTERNS OF IMBALANCE: Too busy to gain perspective on priorities; often feels pressured when making decisions.
POSITIVE QUALITIES: Helps one slow down; promotes harmony in relationships; useful in group dynamic situations, especially when there is a need to find peaceful, common ground.

WILD RHUBARB: *Polygonum alaskanum*
KEY ASPECT: BLOCKED COMMUNICATION
PATTERNS OF IMBALANCE: Mental resistance, inflexibility; mind influenced by the ego; communication between heart and mind blocked or undeveloped.
POSITIVE QUALITIES: Promotes mental flexibility; brings mind into alignment with the heart; encourages balance between the rational and intuitive; ability to discover solutions to problems.

NORTH AMERICAN ESSENCES

ALPINE LILY: *Lilium parvum*
KEY ASPECT: UNGROUNDED FEMININITY
PATTERNS OF IMBALANCE: Sense of being disembodied; alienation of the female body.
POSITIVE QUALITIES: Celebration of femininity; grounded in a bodily experience.

CALENDULA: *Calendula officinalis*
KEY ASPECT: SHARP TONGUE
PATTERNS OF IMBALANCE: Argumentative; lack of receptivity during communication; verbal abuse.
POSITIVE QUALITIES: Creates warmth, receptivity, especially regarding interpersonal communications.

CHAMOMILE: *Matricaria recutita*
KEY ASPECT: OVERSENSITIVITY
PATTERNS OF IMBALANCE: Easily upset, moody and irritable; inability to release emotional tension, especially in the stomach area.
POSITIVE QUALITIES: Helps release tension; fosters serene, sunny-like disposition; emotional balance.

MARIPOSA LILY: *Calochortus leichtlinii*
KEY ASPECT: BONDING ISSUES
PATTERNS OF IMBALANCE: Alienation from one's mother or from mothering; childhood abandonment; situations of adoption or abuse.
POSITIVE QUALITIES: Promotes warmth, nurturing, mother-child bonding; helps heal the inner child.

MORNING GLORY: *Ipomoea purpurea*
KEY ASPECT: DEPLETED NIGHT OWLS
PATTERNS OF IMBALANCE: Addictive or erratic living habits that deplete one's life force, especially in the morning; hung-over feeling.
POSITIVE QUALITIES: Sparkling vital force; feeling awake and refreshed; in touch with life rhythms.

NASTURTIUM: *Matricaria recutita*
KEY ASPECT: INTELLECTUAL IMBALANCE
PATTERNS OF IMBALANCE: Imbalance in certain aspects of life such as education or career, where the demands for intense intellectual activity is dominate.
POSITIVE QUALITIES: Promotes glowing vitality, radiant warmth; balances heart and head.

PRETTY FACE: *Triteleia ixioides*
KEY ASPECT: UNHAPPY WITH PERSONAL APPEARANCE
PATTERNS OF IMBALANCE: Not feeling good about, or overly identified with, one's appearance; feels rejected; born with deformities.
POSITIVE QUALITIES: Helps to get in touch with one's radiant inner beauty and luminosity; self-acceptance in relation to personal appearance despite handicaps or blemishes.

SAINT JOHN'S WORT: *Hypericum perforatum*
KEY ASPECT: OVERLY VULNERABLE
PATTERNS OF IMBALANCE: Sensitive to light; prone to environmental stress; psychic and physical vulnerability; fearful or disturbed dreams; depression; lack of contact with one's innate spirituality.
POSITIVE QUALITIES: Reinstates one's natural illumined consciousness and light-filled awareness.

YARROW: *Achillea millefolium*
KEY ASPECT: SENSITIVITY TO NEGATIVE INFLUENCES
PATTERNS OF IMBALANCE: Extreme vulnerability to others and the environment; easily depleted; overly sensitive to outside influences—especially in an office atmosphere; prone to environmental illness or allergies.
POSITIVE QUALITIES: Promotes inner radiance and strength, compassionate awareness, inclusive sensitivity, beneficent healing forces. (A good essence to keep near your computer.)

AUSTRALIAN BUSH FLOWER ESSENCES

BAUHINIA: *Lysiphyllum cunninghamii*
KEY ASPECT: RIGID ATTITUDES
PATTERNS OF IMBALANCE: Resists change; rigid attitude; gets easily annoyed.
POSITIVE QUALITIES: Helps one embrace new concepts and ideas when there used to be hesitation or reluctance; fosters acceptance and open-mindedness.

BLACK-EYED SUSAN: *Tetratheca ericifolia*
KEY ASPECT: INTERNAL TUNEUP
PATTERNS OF IMBALANCE: Always rushing around; impatient; striving; fills one's life with over commitment; often associated with digestive problems.
POSITIVE QUALITIES: Helps one to slow down, turn inward and be still; creates inner peace to find the still center within; fosters inner guidance; balance to the adrenal glands.

BOAB: *Adansonia gregorii*
KEY ASPECT: NEGATIVE FAMILY PATTERNS
PATTERNS OF IMBALANCE: Takes on negative family thought patterns; repetition of past negativity.
POSITIVE QUALITIES: Helps one release and let go of past, negative experience, and thought patterns within families; useful in relationships to overcome abuse and prejudice; releases deeply held emotions.

BORONIA: *Boronia ledifolia*
KEY ASPECT: STUCK OBSESSIONS
PATTERNS OF IMBALANCE: Obsessive thoughts about events, things, or ideas which become stuck; pines for recently ended relationships; broken-hearted.
POSITIVE QUALITIES: Promotes serenity and focus; clarity of mind and thought. (Combines well with *Bottlebrush* for dealing with an ended relationship.)

BOTTLEBRUSH: *Callistemon linearis*
KEY ASPECT: OVERWHELMED BY MAJOR CHANGE
PATTERNS OF IMBALANCE: Overwhelmed by major life changes: pregnancy, parenthood, new mothers who feel inadequate, menopause, old age; holds on to old habits when approaching the end of a phase; physical symptoms of constipation.
POSITIVE QUALITIES: Promotes serenity, moving forward; assists in bonding between mother and child. (Often needed for only a week.)

BUSH FUCHSIA: *Epacris longiflora*
KEY ASPECT: UNRESOLVED LEARNING ISSUES
PATTERNS OF IMBALANCE: Inability to balance the logical and rational with the intuitive and creative; attention deficit disorder; hyperactivity; dyslexia; switched off, ignores one's gut feeling; clumsy.
POSITIVE QUALITIES: Helps one develop courage and clarity in public speaking; encourages vocalization of one's own convictions; balances left/right hemispheres of the brain; helps in developing intuition.

FIVE CORNERS: *Styphelia laeta*
KEY ASPECT: LOW SELF-ESTEEM
PATTERNS OF IMBALANCE: For low self-esteem; feels crushed, held-in.
POSITIVE QUALITIES: Helps one experience pure love, inner strength, acceptance of self, and the celebration of one's intrinsic beauty; allows the life force to flow through.

LITTLE FLANNEL FLOWER: *Actinotus minor*
KEY ASPECT: SEARCHING FOR THE CHILD WITHIN
PATTERNS OF IMBALANCE: Somber and serious; buttoned-up adults; children who grow up much too quickly, taking on the troubles of the world and grow old before their time; rigid outlook.
POSITIVE QUALITIES: Encourages playfulness, a carefree ability to have fun; allows letting go of inhibitions; spontaneous joy.

MACROCARPA: *Eucalyptus macrocarpa*
KEY ASPECT: BURN-OUT
PATTERNS OF IMBALANCE: Tired, exhausted, sluggish, low immunity; agoraphobia; convalescence.
POSITIVE QUALITIES: Brings energy, inner strength, vitality; renews enthusiasm; has a special affinity to the adrenal glands; a quick pick-me-up.

OLD MAN BANKSIA: *Banksia serrata*
KEY ASPECT: DISHEARTENED BY SETBACKS
PATTERNS OF IMBALANCE: Sluggishness, disheartened, weary, low thyroid activity; frustrated; dependable people who steadily plod on yet hide their weariness.
POSITIVE QUALITIES: Brings renewed energy, enthusiasm; enjoyment of and interest in life.

RED GREVILLEA: *Grevillea speciosa*
KEY ASPECT: STUCK IN THE MUD
PATTERNS OF IMBALANCE: Feels stuck; knows what one wants to achieve but doesn't know how to attain it; too reliant on others.
POSITIVE QUALITIES: Promotes independence and boldness; strength to leave unpleasant situations; extremely effective though changes may not be anticipated.

SHE OAK: *Casuarina glauca*
KEY ASPECT: ISSUES RELATED TO WOMEN
PATTERNS OF IMBALANCE: Female hormonal imbalance; PMS; distress associated with infertility.
POSITIVE QUALITIES: Restores a sense of well-being; helps overcome hormonal imbalances in women; support in overcoming fluid retention.

SPINIFEX: *Triodia species*
KEY ASPECT: PHYSICAL/EMOTIONAL HEALING
PATTERNS OF IMBALANCE: Sense of being a victim of illness; herpes, chlamydia, fine cuts; has no control over illnesses, especially those with persistent and recurring symptoms.
POSITIVE QUALITIES: Empowers one, through emotional understanding, to heal the physical; works well topically on cuts and lesions.

SUNSHINE WATTLE: *Mimosaceae*
KEY ASPECT: LIVES IN THE PAST
PATTERNS OF IMBALANCE: Stuck in the past; feels trapped; has expectations of a grim future.
POSITIVE QUALITIES: Promotes optimism and acceptance of the beauty and joy in the present; helps one open to a bright future; good for dispelling financial worry.

WILD POTATO BUSH: *Solanum quadriloculatum*
KEY ASPECT: HEAVY BURDEN
PATTERNS OF IMBALANCE: Weighed down, encumbered; burdened by the physical body; feels restriction, limitation, and heaviness; desire to step out of old habits but finds it difficult to do.
POSITIVE QUALITIES: Helps one feel free to move forward with renewed enthusiasm; unbinds the feelings of physical restriction and limitation; bodily detox of heavy metals like lead and mercury.

AYURVEDIC ATTARS/ AROMATHERAPEUTIC EXTRACTS

AMBER: *Pinus succinfera*
KEY ASPECT: EMOTIONAL/PHYSICAL BALANCE
PATTERNS OF IMBALANCE: Blood and circulatory system compromised; insomnia.
POSITIVE QUALITIES: Balances the emotions and endocrine system; fosters deeper insight, a quiet and peaceful mind.

FRANKINCENSE: *Boswellia carteri*
KEY ASPECT: STRESSFUL MIND
PATTERNS OF IMBALANCE: Chronic negativity, fear, and distressing psychic forces that stress the mind, body, and spirit.
POSITIVE QUALITIES: Improves memory; stimulates a return to balance and helps one overcome fear.

HONEYSUCKLE: *Lonicera*
KEY ASPECT: ELDER SUPPORT
PATTERNS OF IMBALANCE: Age-related issues such as disinterest; arthritis and diabetic conditions.
POSITIVE QUALITIES: Fosters upliftment; enhances creativity in arts, music, and dance.

JASMINE: *Jasminum grandiflorum*
KEY ASPECT: STRESSFUL SITUATIONS
PATTERNS OF IMBALANCE: Symptoms of sleeplessness, anxiety, and/or depression.
POSITIVE QUALITIES: Promotes a positive outlook; encourages childlike openness and acceptance; aids in balancing mind and body; especially helpful for sleep disorders.

LAVENDER: *Lavandula angustifolia*
KEY ASPECT: UNEASE AND NERVOUSNESS
PATTERNS OF IMBALANCE: Life changes; unease, stress; nervousness and depression.
POSITIVE QUALITIES: Helps create a state of relaxation and restful sleep; dispels negative thought patterns; removes stress from the body and mind.

LILY OF THE VALLEY: *Agapanthus africanus*
KEY ASPECT: RIGIDITY AND LACK OF FOCUS
PATTERNS OF IMBALANCE: Stuck in a state of regression; rigid mental patterns; headaches, obesity issues.
POSITIVE QUALITIES: Stimulates memory and focus of the conscious mind; good for treating mental rigidity.

MUSK: *Mimulus moschatus*
KEY ASPECT: DEPLETED ENERGY
PATTERNS OF IMBALANCE: Decreased vitality; feeling of dizziness.
POSITIVE QUALITIES: Strengthens the entire bodily system; increases one's life force; helps to focus the mind.

MYRRH: *Commiphora myrrha*
KEY ASPECT: TOPICAL ISSUES
PATTERNS OF IMBALANCE: Conditions such as sores, ulcers, and reproductive disorders.
POSITIVE QUALITIES: Helps enhance vision; promotes healing of wounds on both the physical and mental levels.

PATCHOULI: *Pogostemon cablin*
KEY ASPECT: CONCENTRATION AND CONFIDENCE
PATTERNS OF IMBALANCE: Trouble concentrating, often due to stress; lack of confidence; obesity.
POSITIVE QUALITIES: Creates a sense of abundance and self confidence; helps one overcome lethargy, including struggles with weight control.

ROSE: *Rosa damascena*
KEY ASPECT: HEART ISSUES
PATTERNS OF IMBALANCE: Stress-related heart conditions, menopause, eyesight issues, respiratory aliments.
POSITIVE QUALITIES: Opens stifled energies; helps one reconnect with the sense of truth, love, and beauty; an essence of the heart.

SANDALWOOD: *Santalum album*
KEY ASPECT: SPIRITUAL DEPLETION
PATTERNS OF IMBALANCE: For anxiety, depression; fear, especially when facing one's shadow self.
POSITIVE QUALITIES: Promotes calmness, introspection; quiets the senses; spiritual elixir.

WHITE OPIUM: *Papaver somniferum*
KEY ASPECT: LOVE AND MARRIAGE
PATTERNS OF IMBALANCE: Hidden love; inability to express oneself; sensitive nervous system.
POSITIVE QUALITIES: Attracts love, positive vibrations; heightens emotional sensations.

YLANG YLANG: *Cananga odorata*

KEY ASPECT: STRESS AND ANXIETY

PATTERNS OF IMBALANCE: States of anxiety; depression, hypertension, palpitations, and stress.

POSITIVE QUALITIES: A natural sedative; provides relief from anxiety and insomnia; the soothing effect is helpful for problems like rapid breathing or heartbeat; can help normalize blood pressure.

Flower Essence
Flash Cards

An easy way to become familiar with the flower essences highlighted in this book is through the use of flash cards. You can make your own or purchase ours. Download a free sample of six cards. If you would like the full set of ninety-seven cards, you can purchase the digital file. You then have the option of printing them on card or paper stock, single or double-sided, and either in color or black and white. Once you trim them, you'll have a complete, attractively designed set to work with.

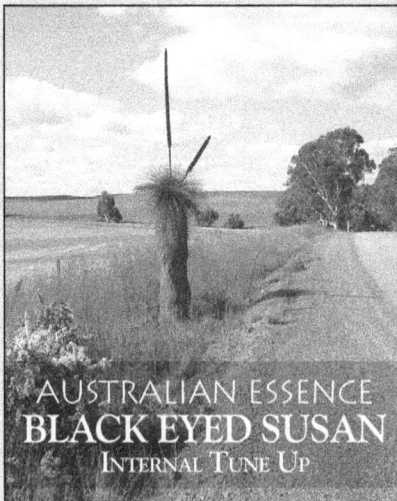

AUSTRALIAN ESSENCE
BLACK EYED SUSAN
INTERNAL TUNE UP

BLACK-EYED SUSAN

PATTERNS OF IMBALANCE: Always rushing around, impatient, striving; filling up one's life with over commitments; often associated with digestive problems.

POSITIVE QUALITIES: Helps one to slow down, turn inward and be still; creates inner peace to find the still center within; fosters inner guidance; balance to the adrenal glands.

www.EssentialFlowerRemedies.com

CROSS REFERENCES
Alphabetized Flower Essence Family Index

Flower Essence Key:
Himalayan Flower Essences (HIM)
Bailey Flower Essences (BAI)
Bach Flower Essences (BAC)
Alaskan Flower Essences (ALK)
Californian Flower Essences (FES)
Australian Flower Essences (AUS)
Aromatherapeutic Extracts (ARM)

Agrimony: BAC
Almond: BAI
Alpine Lily: FES
Amber: ARM
Ashoka Flower: HIM
Aspen: BAC
Bauhinia: AUS
Beech: BAC
Bistort: BAI
Black Spruce: ALK
Black-Eyed Susan: AUS
Boab: AUS
Boronia: AUS
Bottlebrush: AUS
Bush Fuchsia: AUS
Calendula: FES
Centaury: BAC
Cerato: BAC
Chamomile: FES
Cherry Plum: BAC
Chestnut Bud: BAC
Chicory: BAC
Clematis: BAC
Crab Apple: BAC
Elm: BAC

Five Corners: AUS
Foxglove: ALK
Frankincense: ARM
Fuji Cherry: BAI
Gentian: BAC
Gorse: BAC
Heath Bedstraw: BAI
Heather: BAC
Holly: BAC
Honeysuckle: ARM
Honeysuckle: BAC
Hornbeam: BAC
Impatiens: BAC
Jasmine: ARM
Lamb's Quarter: ALK
Larch: BAC
Lavender: ARM
Lily of the Valley: ARM
Little Flannel Flower: AUS
Lotus: HIM
Macrocarpa: AUS
Mariposa Lily: FES
Mimulus: BAC
Monkshood: ALK
Morning Glory: FES
Musk: ARM
Mustard: BAC
Myrrh: ARM
Nasturtium: FES
Neem: HIM
Oak: BAC
Old Man Banksia: AUS
Olive: BAC
Opium Poppy: ALK

Oriental Poppy: BAI
Parrot Tree Flower: HIM
Patchouli: ARM
Peacock Flower: HIM
Pine: BAC
Pretty Face: FES
Red Chestnut: BAC
Red Grevillea: AUS
Rescue Remedy (Rock Rose, Cherry
    Plum, Clematis, Impatiens, and
    Star of Bethlehem): BAC
Rock Rose: BAC
Rock Water: BAC
Rose: ARM
Saint John's Wort: FES
Sandalwood: ARM
Scleranthus: BAC
She Oak: AUS
Solomon's Seal: BAI
Spinifex: AUS

Star of Bethlehem: BAC
Sunshine Wattle: AUS
Sweet Chestnut: BAC
Teakwood Flower: HIM
Valerian: FES
Vervain: BAC
Vine: BAC
Walnut: BAC
Water Violet: BAC
White Chestnut: BAC
White Dead Nettle: BAI
White Opium: ARM
Wild Oat: BAC
Wild Potato Bush: AUS
Wild Rhubarb: ALK
Wild Rose: BAC
Willow: BAC
Yarrow: FES
Ylang Ylang: ARM

The Seven Bach Flower Groups

Despondency or Despair
Crab Apple, Elm,
Larch, Oak, Pine,
Star of Bethlehem,
Sweet Chestnut,
Willow

Fear
Aspen, Cherry Plum,
Mimulus,
Red Chestnut,
Rock Rose

Insufficient Interest in Present Circumstances
Chestnut Bud,
Clematis, Honeysuckle,
Mustard, Olive,
White Chestnut,
Wild Rose

Loneliness
Heather, Impatiens,
Water Violet

Overcare for Welfare of Others
Beech, Chicory,
Rock Water,
Vervain, Vine,

Oversensitivity to Influences and Ideas
Agrimony, Centaury,
Holly, Walnut,

Uncertainty
Cerato, Gentian, Gorse,
Hornbeam, Scleranthus,
Wild Oat

Flower Essence Reference by Issue

This is a simple guide and starting point. Remember, essences are always specific to the person and the issue(s) one is dealing with at the moment. Someone taking Aspen for anxiety may be using it for an unknown fear, while someone taking Fuji Cherry may be using it for the anxiety of getting caught up in a life event. For detailed information about each essence, refer to the Selection Guide beginning on page 106.

Abuse - FES: Calendula, Mariposa Lily, Morning Glory; AUS: Boab,
    Black-Eyed Susan

Addiction and Dependency - HIM: Peacock Flower; BAI: Oriental Poppy,
    White Dead Nettle; FES: Morning Glory; ALK: Opium Poppy;
    AUS: Boab, Red Grevillea

Adrenal Issues - AUS: Black-Eyed Susan, Macrocarpa; FES: Chamomile

Anger - BAC: Beech, Holly
        AROMATHERAPY: Jasmine, Patchouli, Rose, Ylang Ylang

Anxiety - BAC: Agrimony, Aspen, Cherry Plum, Gorse, Mimulus, Mustard,
    Red Chestnut, Rock Rose, Sweet Chestnut; BAI: Fuji Cherry;
    FES: Chamomile
        AROMATHERAPY: Jasmine, Lavender, Sandalwood, Ylang Ylang

Apathy - BAC: Wild Rose; HIM: Teakwood Flower; FES: Nasturtium;
    AUS: Bush Fuchsia, Old Man Banksia
        AROMATHERAPY: Honeysuckle

Attachment Issues - BAC: Chicory, Honeysuckle, Red Chestnut,
    Water Violet; AUS: Bottlebrush; FES: Mariposa Lily

Autism Issues - BAC: Chicory, Clematis, Impatiens; FES: Mariposa Lily,
    Saint John's Wort, Yarrow
        AROMATHERAPY: Lavender

Bonding - BAC: Holly, Water Violet; FES: Black-Eyed Susan, Mariposa Lily;
    ALK: Lamb's Quarter; AUS: Bottlebrush
        AROMATHERAPY: Sandalwood

Burned Out - BAC: Hornbeam, Elm, Oak, Olive; AUS: Macrocarpa,
    Old Man Banksia, Wild Potato Bush; FES: Morning Glory; Nasturtium,
    Yarrow
        AROMATHERAPY: Patchouli

Communication Difficulties - BAC: Heather, Impatiens, Larch;
    HIM: Parrot Tree Flower, Teakwood Flower; AUS: Bush Fuchsia;
    FES: Calendula; ALK: Wild Rhubarb
        AROMATHERAPY: Patchouli, White Opium

Concentration (Lack of) - BAC: Clematis, White Chestnut;

HIM: Lotus; BAI: Fuji Cherry, Solomon's Seal, White Dead Nettle
AROMATHERAPY: Patchouli

Confusion - BAC: Centaury, Cerato, Clematis, Scleranthus,
White Chestnut, Wild Oat; HIM: Teakwood Flower; AUS: Red Grevillea
AROMATHERAPY: Musk, Honeysuckle

Depression - BAC: Gentian, Gorse, Larch, Mustard, Oak, Pine; BAI: Bistort;
FES: Saint John's Wort
AROMATHERAPY: Jasmine, Lavender, Sandalwood, Ylang Ylang

Despair - BAC: Cherry Plum, Gentian, Gorse, Mustard, Sweet Chestnut,
Willow
AROMATHERAPY: Honeysuckle, Jasmine

Discouragement - BAC: Elm, Gentian, Wild Oat; AUS: Sunshine Wattle,
Old Man Banksia, Wild Potato Bush
AROMATHERAPY: Jasmine, Lavender

Distracted Mind - BAC: Clematis, Scleranthus, White Chestnut;
HIM: Lotus; BAI: Solomon's Seal, White Dead Nettle; ALK: Valerian
AROMATHERAPY: Musk

Dogmatic - BAC: Vine; AUS: Bauhinia
AROMATHERAPY: Lavender

Dyslexia - BAC: Chestnut Bud, Larch, White Chestnut;
HIM: Parrot Tree Flower; AUS: Bush Fuchsia

Elder Aid - BAC: Honeysuckle, Wild Rose; HIM: Ashoka Flower,
Teakwood Flower; AUS: Bottlebrush
AROMATHERAPY: Honeysuckle, Rose

Exhaustion - BAC: Elm, Hornbeam, Oak, Olive; HIM: Lotus,
Peacock Flower, Teakwood Flower; AUS: Macrocarpa, Old Man Banksia,
Wild Potato Bush; ALK: Opium Poppy; FES: Morning Glory, Nasturtium,
Yarrow
AROMATHERAPY: Frankincense, Musk, Sandalwood

Fear - BAC: Aspen, Cherry Plum, Larch, Mimulus, Red Chestnut, Rock Rose;
ALK: Foxglove; AUS: Black-Eyed Susan
AROMATHERAPY: Frankincense, Honeysuckle, Sandalwood

Focus (Lack of) - BAC: Chestnut Bud, Clematis, White Chestnut, Wild Oat;
HIM: Lotus; BAI: Heath Bedstraw, Solomon's Seal, White Dead Nettle;
AUS: Black-Eyed Susan, Boronia
AROMATHERAPY: Lily of the Valley, Musk, Patchouli

Frustration - BAC: Agrimony, Beech, Gentian, Vervain; BAI: Bistort

Grief - BAC: Gorse, Honeysuckle, Star of Bethlehem; HIM: Ashoka Flower;
FES: Chamomile; AUS: Boronia
AROMATHERAPY: Honeysuckle, Sandalwood

Guilt - BAC: Centaury, Pine

Heart Issues - BAC: Crab Apple; HIM: Neem; ALK: Foxglove, Wild Rhubarb
    AROMATHERAPY: Honeysuckle, ROSE, YLANG YLANG

Hormonal Issues - BAC: Crab Apple; AUS: She Oak, Old Man Banksia
    AROMATHERAPY: Amber

Humor (Lack of) - BAC: Rock Water, Wild Rose;
    AUS: Little Flannel Flower, Old Man Banksia; FES: Chamomile
    AROMATHERAPY: Honeysuckle, Jasmine

Hyperactivity - BAC: White Chestnut; AUS: Black-Eyed Susan,
    Bush Fuchsia; FES: Morning Glory, Valerian; BAI: Solomon's Seal,
    White Dead Nettle
    AROMATHERAPY: Jasmine, Lavender

Imbalance - BAC: Clematis, Scleranthus; AUS: She Oak
    AROMATHERAPY: Musk

Impatience - BAC: Impatiens; BAI: Solomon's Seal; AUS: Black-Eyed Susan
    AROMATHERAPY: Patchouli

Indecision - BAC: Scleranthus, Wild Oat; AUS: Red Grevillea
    AROMATHERAPY: Amber, Musk

Intolerance - BAC: Beech, Impatiens, Vervain, Vine; AUS: Bauhinia, Boab
    AROMATHERAPY: Jasmine

Intuition (Lack of) - BAC: Cerato; HIM: Lotus, Neem; BAI: Almond;
    AUS: Wild Rhubarb; ALK: Foxglove, Valerian; AUS: Bush Fuchsia
    AROMATHERAPY: Amber, Myrrh, Sandalwood

Irritability - BAC: Beech, Impatiens, Pine; HIM: Teakwood Flower;
    FES: Chamomile; AUS: Bauhinia
    AROMATHERAPY: Sandalwood

Isolation - BAC: Water Violet; HIM: Ashoka Flower; ALK: Monkshood

Jealousy - BAC: Chicory, Holly

Judgemental - BAC: Beech, Vervain; HIM: Neem

Lack of Direction - BAC: Scleranthus, Wild Oat; AUS: Red Grevillea

Learning Disabilities - BAC: Chestnut Bud, Clematis, White Chestnut;
    HIM: Parrot Tree Flower; AUS: Bush Fuchsia, Five Corners

Learning (Repeat Mistakes) - BAC: Chestnut Bud; AUS: Boab;
    ALK: Opium Poppy

Life Changes - BAC: Walnut; HIM: Ashoka Flower
    BAI: Bistort, Fuji Cherry, Heath Bedstraw; AUS: Bauhinia, Bottlebrush
    AROMATHERAPY: Lavender

Loneliness - BAC: Agrimony, Heather, Water Violet
    AROMATHERAPY: Frankincense, Rose

Mood Swings - BAC: Scleranthus; FES: Chamomile; AUS: Bauhinia

Negativity - BAC: Beech, Holly, Honeysuckle, Pine, Willow; AUS: Boab
    AROMATHERAPY: Frankincense, Jasmine, Lavender

Nervousness - BAC: Agrimony, Impatiens, White Chestnut;
    FES: Chamomile; BAI: Solomon's Seal, White Dead Nettle
    AROMATHERAPY: Lavender, White Opium

Nightmares - BAC: Aspen, Crab Apple, Rock Rose, Rescue Remedy;
    FES: Saint John's Wort

Obsession - BAC: Agrimony, Crab Apple, Rock Water, White Chestnut;
    HIM: Peacock Flower; AUS: Boronia; Oriental Poppy,
    White Dead Nettle

Overwhelmed - BAC: Centaury, Cherry Plum, Elm, Hornbeam, Oak;
    BAI: Fuji Cherry, Solomon's Seal; AUS: Black-Eyed Susan,
    Bottlebrush
    AROMATHERAPY: Lavender, Rose

Past Issues - BAC: Honeysuckle, Star of Bethlehem; BAI: Almond,
    Heath Bedstraw; ALK: Black Spruce, Opium Poppy; AUS: Boab,
    Bottlebrush, Sunshine Wattle, Wild Potato Bush
    AROMATHERAPY: Jasmine

Perfectionism - BAC: Agrimony, Beech, Vervain; AUS: Boronia

Possessiveness - BAC: Chicory, Red Chestnut

Procrastination - BAC: Hornbeam, Scleranthus; AUS: Bottlebrush,
    Red Grevillea

Recuperation - BAC: Crab Apple, Gorse, Hornbeam, Olive; HIM: Lotus,
    Peacock Flower; AUS: Macrocarpa, Spinifex
    AROMATHERAPY: Frankincense, Myrrh

Resentment - BAC: Holly, Willow

Restlessness: - BAC: Scleranthus, Wild Oat; HIM: Heath Bedstraw, Lotus;
    BAI: Solomon's Seal; AUS: Black-Eyed Susan, White Dead Nettle,
    Wild Potato Bush; FES: Morning Glory, Chamomile; ALK: Valerian
    AROMATHERAPY: JAsmine, Lavender, Ylang Ylang

Rigidity - BAC: Beech, Rock Water, Vine, Water Violet;
    BAI: Heath Bedstraw; AUS: Bauhinia, Little Flannel Flower;
    ALK: Wild Rhubarb
    AROMATHERAPY: Honeysuckle, Lily of the Valley

Sadness - BAC: Gentian, Gorse, Honeysuckle, Mustard, Pine;
    HIM: Ashoka Flower; AUS: Old Man Banksia
    AROMATHERAPY: Honeysuckle, Sandalwood

Self-Esteem/Image Issues - BAC: Centaury, Cerato, Crab Apple, Larch;
    HIM: Parrot Tree Flower; AUS: Five Corners, Bush Fuchsia;
    FES: Pretty Face

AROMATHERAPY: Patchouli

Selfishness - BAC: Chicory, Heather, Holly

Sensitive (Overly) - BAC: Walnut; AUS: Red Grevillea,
FES: Chamomile, Saint John's Wort, Yarrow
AROMATHERAPY: Honeysuckle

Shyness - BAC: Larch, Mimulus; AUS: Five Corners

Sleep Disturbances - BAC: Aspen, Mimulus, White Chestnut, Wild Oat;
BAI: Fuji Cherry, Solomon's Seal; AUS: Boronia; FES: Chamomile,
Morning Glory
AROMATHERAPY: Amber, Jasmine, Lavender, Ylang Ylang

Sluggishness - BAC: Clematis, Hornbeam, Wild Rose; AUS: Macrocarpa,
Old Man Banksia; FES: Morning Glory
AROMATHERAPY: Honeysuckle, Lily of the Valley, Patchouli

Skin Problems - BAC: Crab Apple; AUS: Spinifex
AROMATHERAPY: Musk, Myrrh

Speech Issues - HIM: Parrot Tree Flower; AUS: Bush Fuchsia, Red Grevillea;
FES: Calendula

Spiritual Disconnect - BAC: Aspen; BAI: Almond, Fuji Cherry;
ALK: Black Spruce, Monkshood
AROMATHERAPY: Sandalwood

Stress - BAC: Mimulus, Impatiens, Rescue Remedy; BAI: Fuji Cherry,
Solomon's Seal; FES: Chamomile; ALK: Foxglove
AROMATHERAPY: Frankincense, Jasmine, Patchouli, Ylang Ylang,
White Opium

Trauma - BAC: Cherry Plum, Rescue Remedy, Rock Rose, Star of Bethlehem,
Sweet Chestnut; HIM: Ashoka Flower
AROMATHERAPY: Honeysuckle, Lavender, Rose, Ylang Ylang

Trust (Lack of) - BAC: Aspen, Cerato, Holly, Red Chestnut;
FES: Mariposa Lily

Unbalanced (Heart and Mind) - HIM: Neem; ALK: Lamb's Quarter

Weakness - BAC: Centaury; BAI: Solomon's Seal; FES: Saint John's Wort;
AUS: Red Grevillea
AROMATHERAPY: Jasmine, Lavender, Ylang Ylang

Women's Issues - BAC: Centaury, Crab Apple, Red Chestnut, Walnut;
HIM: Ashoka Flower; AUS: Bottlebrush, Macrocarpa, She Oak;
FES: Alpine Lily, Mariposa Lily, Pretty Face
AROMATHERAPY: Amber, Myrrh, Patchouli

Worry - BAC: Agrimony, Red Chestnut, White Chestnut;
FES: Saint John's Wort; AUS: Sunshine Wattle
AROMATHERAPY: Jasmine, Ylang Ylang

HOW TO PREPARE DROPS AND CREAMS

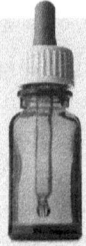

The Dosage Bottle

- Fill a one-ounce (30 ml) amber or blue glass dropper bottle nearly full of purified or chlorine-free water.
- Add a small amount of preservative: brandy, whiskey, vegetable glycerin, or shiso—about ⅛ teaspoon per bottle. More preservative should be added if the dosage bottle is to be used slowly over a number of months or if you are traveling to a place with high temperatures or extreme humidity.
- Add the correct amount of drops to your bottle, according to the recommendation of each flower essences stock bottle. Try to limit the essence combinations to no more than seven, eight tops.
- Label and date the bottle.
- After all the essence(s) are added to the dropper bottle, shake bottle slightly in order to reenergize the essences before using.
- Place 2-4 drops directly under the tongue.
- Another way to administer the essences is to add 4 drops to a half glass of water or small water bottle. Gently mix or shake each time before sipping.
- A common dosage is four times a day. This bottle will last about three weeks to one month. At that time, you may want to re-assess the combination, make another bottle, or change the ingredients.
- Glass droppers and mister bottles are best, since plastic may adversely affect the essences' subtle qualities. Either use new glass bottles or sterilize old ones to maintain cleanliness and clarity of the vibrational patterns.
- Keep the bottles out of direct sunlight and avoid exposure to heat and strong scents.

Spray Bottles or Misters:
This is recommended for babies, children, and pets. It is also ideal for misting rooms.

- Prepare exactly as you would a dropper bottle, but use a bottle with a mister top.
- Gently shake the mister bottle before each application to reestablish its potency.
- Mist at least 30" from the person, or straight up into the room.

How to Use in a Bath or Foot Spa

- Double the amount of drops recommended for the particular essence you are using. Drop essences directly into a bathtub filled with warm water.
- Stir the water in a figure-eight motion for a minute or two to re-potentize the essences.
- After your bath, pat your skin gently dry. To continue to absorb the subtle flower essence qualities, rest after the bath or take a bath just before sleep.
- *For a foot spa*: add the recommended dose of each essence to one cup of all-natural mineral or dead sea salts. Place in a sealed container. You can also include a few drops of any soothing aromatherapeutic extract to this mixture. Add 3-4 tablespoons of essence salts to a warm bucket of water or a foot spa. Stir to dissolve and re-potentize. Soak your feet for at least 15 minutes and gently pat dry.

How to Use Topically in a Cream Base

- Shea Butter or Aloe Vera are good mediums. Avoid using a base that has a lot of extra ingredients or any kind of perfume. Many cream bases contain a preservative and can stay fresh for up to six months. Labeling and dating each preparation is important. If the cream begins to smell, it's time to replace the remedies using a fresh cream base.
- Add the correct amount of drops recommended by the flower essences manufacturer. You may also add a few drops of pure Ayurvedic attars or aromatherapeutic extracts. Be careful not to add too much or it will overtake the cream mixture.
- To apply: dab on the inside of each wrist, the crook of your arm, or on each temple. You may repeat this application as often as needed but three-four times a day is a typical daily dose.
- For sleep issues, you may repeat as often as needed, even re-applying it an hour before waking. There are no side effects, nor will you wake up feeling tired or groggy.
- You may also use the creams during massage, meditation, yoga, acupressure, acupuncture, or with chiropractic treatments. It is especially helpful and soothing for a baby massage.

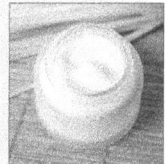

FLOWER ESSENCE DIAGNOSTIC FORM©

Copy this form so that you can use it again and again.
You can also download a PDF copy from: www.EssentialFlowerRemedies.com

WORK THROUGH ISSUES TO DETERMINE THE APPROPRIATE ESSENCE(S).

Descriptive Issue(s):

PROFILE
Primary Issues:
Emotion/State of Mind:
Manifests As:
Positive Aspects:

TREATMENT
Bach:

Himalayan:

Bailey:

Alaskan:

Californian (FES):

Australian Bush:

Ayurvedic Attar/Aromatherapy:

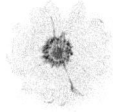

INDEX

L

lack of direction 131
law of similars 2
learning disabilities 131
learning (repeat mistakes) 131
Leonard Cohen 83
Leonardo da Vinci 61
letting go 26, 53, 64, 67, 108, 113, 120, 121
life changes 26, 35, 63, 64, 66, 107, 121, 124, 131
loneliness 24, 28, 128, 131
low thyroid 122
Lucy Cornelssen xvi, xvii
Luther Burbank 1

M

major changes 115, 121
Martin Buxbaum 41
Masaru-Emoto 15.
    See also Dr. Emoto
Maurice Maeterlinck 21
meditation xvi, 21, 22, 47, 49, 53, 72, 106, 135
menopause 73, 115, 121, 125
Michel Foucault 13
moody 25, 35, 53, 58, 61, 68, 82, 114, 118, 131

N

negativity 5, 7, 15, 17, 25, 27, 33, 45, 66, 76, 78, 104, 107, 120, 123, 124, 132
nervousness 28, 124, 132
nervous system 17, 107, 125
Nicholas Culpeper 12
nightmares 89, 109, 132
nonjudgemental xvii
North American Essences xi, 51, 85, 118. *See also* FES
    Alpine Lily 35, 118, 133
    Black-Eyed Susan 129
    Calendula 118, 129, 133
    Chamomile 35, 52, 53, 68, 70, 74, 76, 82, 92, 118, 129, 130, 131, 132, 133
    Clematis 129
    Mariposa Lily 35, 42, 119, 129, 133
    Morning Glory 34, 80, 99, 119, 129, 130, 131, 132, 133
    Nasturtium 70, 119, 129, 130
    Pretty Face 51, 119, 132, 133
    Saint John's Wort 74, 81, 119, 129, 130, 132, 133
    Valerian 131
    Wild Rhubarb 129
    Yarrow 120, 129, 130, 133
no side effects 2, 6, 39, 102, 135

O

obesity 124, 125
obsession 25, 63, 65, 79, 83, 108, 110, 121, 132
online resources 21, 105
optimism 28, 45, 116, 123
overprotective 5, 71
overresponsibility 69
oversensitivity 24, 67, 81, 118, 128, 133
overwhelmed 55, 65, 121, 132

P

panic 28, 42, 81, 83, 84, 114
Paracelsus 10, 11, 12
past 5, 23, 42, 63, 64, 66, 80, 107, 110, 112, 114, 117, 120, 123
past issues 132
Patanjali xv
perfectionism 83, 132
pessimism 112
Petite Fleur 87
pity 28, 116
placebo 4, 41, 86
possessiveness 35, 65, 71, 110, 132

ABOUT THE AUTHOR

In 1979, while working on a publication project in South India, Joan Greenblatt met Lucy Cornelssen, a German writer and mystic. Lucy, who was ninety-two years young at the time, enjoyed great health. She introduced Joan to, and later mentored her in, the unique healing abilities of flower essences. After returning to the States, Joan studied with the *Dr. Edward Bach Centre* and later took Advanced Worldwide Flower Essences and Aromatherapy courses from *the School of Natural Health Sciences*, were she graduated with honors. She holds diplomas in all three protocols.

Throughout the over thirty years that Joan has continued to consult as a flower essence practitioner, she found that even after successful treatment for a specific issue, people still faced a number of general challenges such as sleep, stress, diet, confidence, fear, hormonal challenges, etc.—issues that often appeared in their lives from time to time. Several years ago, Joan developed an original collection of flower essence combinations under the name *Flower Essence Healing Crèmes.* She uses a cream base to store the essences, which introduces them quickly and efficiently through surface veins in the skin, thus providing a time-release like effect. Joan has incorporated a variety of flower essences from different parts of the world, as well as subtle Ayurvedic attars and aromatherapeutic extracts, to enhance each unique formula.

Joan, along with her husband, Matthew, are the founders of the nonprofit organization Inner Directions. Her creative activities also include award-winning graphic design. Joan and her husband reside in Southern California.

Aperion Books
Book Publishing for the Digital Age

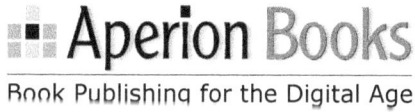

Aperion Books is dedicated to producing high quality publications that help people facilitate positive change in their lives. We specialize in publishing titles on spirituality, wellness, and personal growth.

Our unique Collaborative Publishing Program is specifically designed to help writers and authors expand their personal and professional horizons through creatively designed books that are distributed to national wholesalers and leading retailers.

NOTES

Use this space for taking notes
as you go through the book.

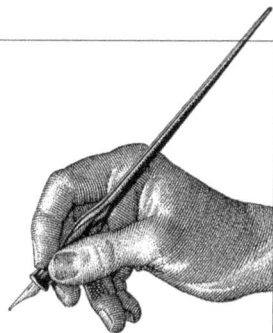

www.ingramcontent.com/pod-product-compliance
Lightning Source LLC
Chambersburg PA
CBHW021828020426
42334CB00014B/538